DISEASES
from
OUTER SPACE
Our Cosmic Destiny
Second Edition

A revised and extended second edition of Hoyle and Wickramasinghe's 1979 classic *Diseases from Space*.

DISEASES
from
OUTER SPACE
Our Cosmic Destiny

Second Edition

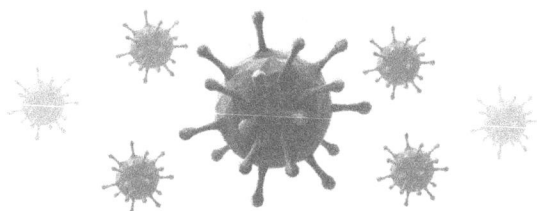

Chandra Wickramasinghe
University of Buckingham, UK

W **World Scientific**

NEW JERSEY · LONDON · SINGAPORE · BEIJING · SHANGHAI · HONG KONG · TAIPEI · CHENNAI · TOKYO

Published by

World Scientific Publishing Co. Pte. Ltd.

5 Toh Tuck Link, Singapore 596224

USA office: 27 Warren Street, Suite 401-402, Hackensack, NJ 07601

UK office: 57 Shelton Street, Covent Garden, London WC2H 9HE

Library of Congress Cataloging-in-Publication Data

Names: Wickramasinghe, Chandra, 1939–   author.

Title: Diseases from outer space : our cosmic destiny /
    Chandra Wickramasinghe, University of Buckingham, UK.

Other titles: Diseases from space

Description: Second edition. | New Jersey : World Scientific, [2020] | Revised edition of:
    Diseases from space / Fred Hoyle, Chandra Wickramasinghe by Harper & Row, 1980. |
    Includes bibliographical references and index.

Identifiers: LCCN 2020028768 | ISBN 9789811222122 (hardcover) |
    ISBN 9789811222139 (ebook)

Subjects: LCSH: Space medicine. | Communicable diseases--Etiology. |
    Diseases--Causes and theories of causation.

Classification: LCC RC1137 .H69 2020 | DDC 616.9/80214--dc23

LC record available at https://lccn.loc.gov/2020028768

British Library Cataloguing-in-Publication Data

A catalogue record for this book is available from the British Library.

First published in Great Britain by J. M. Dent & Sons Ltd. 1979

Copyright © Fred Hoyle and Chandra Wickramasinghe 1979

Published by Sphere Books Ltd. 1981

For any available supplementary material, please visit
https://www.worldscientific.com/worldscibooks/10.1142/11879#t=suppl

Foreword

It is now just over 40 years since the first edition of this monumental book first appeared in London, published by J. M. Dent & Sons Ltd. It is monumental as it ranks with the greatest books of all time, along with those by Aristotle, Plato, Copernicus, Galileo, Kepler and Newton. So, if you do nothing else in your life, I recommend that all intelligent men and women read *Diseases from Outer Space — Our Cosmic Destiny* before they die. I unabashedly herald this book as the greatest in human history. Read it and in your quiet moment you will agree with me.

Why so? For Sir Fred Hoyle and Professor N. Chandra Wickramasinghe, this was only one of several landmark books and compendia they published together (and since Fred's death in 2001, continued at a remarkable pace by Chandra himself). It was the second in what they called their "Trilogy" — the first *Life Cloud* (1978), and the third *Evolution from Space* (1981). While the entire H–W oeuvre will be read and re-read while intelligent life exists on Earth, this book earns a special place at the very top of the Pantheon — it encapsulates all the key principles of Panspermia which now guides the new scientific discipline of Astrobiology — which they founded in one of the greatest scientific journeys and collaborations of all time. It is unequivocally the "University 101" level primer, not only for studies in the detail of the origins and evolution of life on Earth, in microbiology, virology and immunology, but also, most importantly to the study of epidemiology itself — the origin and spread of newly emerging infectious diseases. It also puts on display the significance of the carbon-rich comets in marking out the history of life on Earth. They are the universal incubators of living systems in our Solar

Systems and beyond. Comets are thus the primary vehicles for the spread of life forms for long space journeys that could last a billion years before delivery of its living cargo to a congenial cosmic niche, such as the Earth. Their cargos are compact travellers that reflect the living principle that "..from little things big things grow.." — spores, bacteria, viruses, seeds, microorganisms and fungi, fertilised eggs, and mature yet microscopic plants and animals. Many will most likely be cryopreserved on the outer layers of such bolides as the temperature of deep space is only a few degrees above absolute zero (about 2.7 Kelvin or –270.45 Celsius and –454.81 Fahrenheit).

Thus, by implication, all living systems on Earth are "Space hardy" — they not only survived the rigours of long distance-time space travel *per se* (in their protective vehicles and matrices) but also the fiery impact events themselves, the meteorites streaking across the sky each night.

But it has been the arrival of COVID-19 in late 2019 in Wuhan, China which has roiled the world with devastating economic force. Compared to past pandemics the virus itself is a mild dose of the "cosmic" common cold.

While he was alive, Fred and Chandra often reflected on what it would take for the mainstream scientific community to take Panspermia seriously, viz. the continuous seeding of living systems to Earth from the Cosmos. The arrival of COVID-19 I think fits that bill.

Edward J. Steele
Melbourne, April 2020

Contents

List of Figures

Acknowledgements

At various stages of this work we have had the benefit of discussions and technological advice from many colleagues. Our particular thanks go to Sir Christopher Andrewes and Dr Sylvia Reed of the Common Cold Research Institute, Salisbury, Drs C. W. L. Howells, P. Mann and M. S. Pereira of the Public Health Laboratory Services, Prof. J. F. Watkins and Dr D. Westmorland of the Department of Medical Microbiology, University Hospital of Wales, Prof. V. M. Zhdanov, V. Ivanovsky of the Institute of Virology, Moscow, Prof. P. Walcot, Department of Classics, University College, Cardiff, Prof. S. N. Wickramasinghe, Saint Mary's Hospital, London, and Dr J. Briscoe, Medical Officer, Eton College, and Dr P. de la Motte, Ministry of Health, Sri Lanka. We also wish to record our thanks to headmasters, school doctors, matrons and nurses in over four hundred schools throughout England and Wales for their painstaking help and co-operation in our influenza survey.

The authors and publisher are grateful to the following for permission to quote extracts:

Weidenfeld (Publishers) Ltd for permission to quote from *The Common Cold* by Sir Christopher Andrewes;

The Folio Society and K. R. Mackenzie for permission to quote from his translation of Virgil's *Georgics*;

Penguin Books for permission to quote from E. V. Rieu's translation of Homer's *Iliad*;

Dr John Chadwick for permission to quote from *Hipprocratic Writings*, Penguin Books, 1978;

The New England Journal of Medicine, 6 May 1976, for permission to quote from an article by Dr Louis Weinstein.

1

Descent from Space

In *Diseases from Space* we shall be presenting arguments and facts which support the idea that the viruses and bacteria responsible for the infectious diseases of plants and animals arrive at the Earth from space. Furthermore, we shall argue that apart from their harmful effect, these same viruses and bacteria have been responsible in the past for the origin and evolution of life on the Earth. In our view, all aspects of the basic biochemistry of life come from outside the Earth.

Bacteria are living cells of a comparatively simple kind that exist and multiply by using similar nutrients to other more complex cells, such as those which make up our own bodies. Not all bacteria are harmful. Some have little or no interaction with plants and animals, while others serve useful functions. Bacteria in the gut of a sheep break down cellulose in the grass eaten by the sheep into its constituent sugar (glucose) molecules, and the sugar then becomes the animal's source of food energy. Unlike the sheep and the cow, we humans cannot usefully eat grass because we do not carry the right kind of bacteria in our stomachs. The useful bacteria that animals carry inside them maintain their numbers at more or less steady levels, whereas harmful bacteria seek to multiply their numbers uncontrollably. When this happens inside us the consequence is a drain on the materials which should go towards maintaining the normal cells of our bodies. Moreover, the bacteria themselves exude chemical wastes that may poison us severely, as happens for instance in the disease of botulism.

Although bacteria can cause extremely serious infections — pneumonia, tuberculosis and bubonic plague are other examples —

1

their mode of attack is more straightforward than the attack of viruses; and as a general rule, medical science has had greater success in coping with bacteria than with viruses. Viruses multiply by, entering and destroying living cells, not by making use of comparatively simple materials. Whereas the harm that some bacteria do to us is in a sense a by-product of their activity, the attack of viruses on our cells is direct, and seemingly quite deliberate. Plainly, viruses have a close and intricate chemical connection with living cells. This raises the question of how a virus that evolved in some place other than the Earth could have become equipped with the ability to attack cells here on the Earth. The question is sharpened by the fact that specific viruses only attack specific kinds of cell. How, one may wonder, could a virus coming from a comet have foreseen the kind of living cell it was going to encounter after its arrival here on Earth?

There is obviously no direct answer to this question, but a decisive answer can be reached by turning the question around. The invading virus cannot know in advance about its terrestrial host, but the host can know about the virus, for the reason that terrestrial host cells have had a vast experience of invading viruses, an experience extending back in time over thousands of millions of years.

This experience could well have been imprinted in our genes and in the structure of our cells. The possibility of the host cell being adapted through long experience to receive certain types of bacteria and viruses, types for which the host cell has past knowledge, is entirely viable in theory. The reasons why critics of our point of view seem always to overlook this quite simple reversal of the problem lie undoubtedly in the deep-rooted conviction we all have that disease is bad for us. So it is for the individual, but not necessarily for the species as a whole. In Chapter 10 we shall argue that disease is essential to every species, because it is from invading viruses and bacteria that ultimately we derive all important changes, all worthwhile advances in our evolution, all improvements (paradoxical as it may seem) in our physique and in our mental capacity.

We turn now to a second very relevant question. Every cell, whether the simple forms of bacteria or the more complex cells of plants and animals, works on the same chemical system. So too do viruses. The system is exceedingly complex. In the past it was fashionable to compare the chemistry of life to a piece of precision machinery, like a watch, although no watch remotely approaches the subtlety of biochemistry in its construction. Now if the Earth derives its bacteria and viruses from not just one external body but from many, we have to suppose that exactly the same biochemistry exists in all such bodies. The question then arises of how this can be. Would one not expect the chemistry of life to evolve in different ways in different places — for example, through the use of somewhat different amino acids in the construction of proteins? Our answer to these questions is an emphatic no. One would expect all systems to be the same, for the reason that, if external bodies seed the Earth with life, they can also seed each other.

The most important quality of biology lies in its ability to increase numbers explosively. During the interval of two to three days between 'catching' a cold and the moment when you first begin. to sneeze violently, the common cold virus multiplies its number inside you about ten thousand millionfold. And if the virus could keep on growing at the same rate for three weeks instead of three days, the eventual mass of it would exceed the combined masses of all the stars in the Milky Way. This means that in early days, when many chemical systems in many comets (there are thousands of millions of comets) were competing to produce the first working biological system, when they were shedding and scattering their products among each other, the first system to 'make it' scooped the pool. It was a case of winner takes all. The explosive power of biology forced biochemical unity on the solar system.

As a matter of personal history, we did not arrive at our ideas at all light-heartedly. Over the past ten years, astronomers have discovered more than one hundred and fifty organic molecules present in the gas which lies between the stars, particularly in dense blobs of gas out of which new stars are continually being born. As well as the gas between the stars, there are also myriads of small solid particles, often called grains. We discovered two years ago that the neat emission properties of these grains are uncannily similar to the known heat properties of the commonest of all biological substances, the material cellulose, which gives strength to the stalks of ground plants and to the wood of trees. This work, which was discussed in more detail in our previous book *Lifecloud*, is reviewed in the present book in Appendix 1.

These facts and clues forced us to ask ourselves whether the solar system might not have acquired a first supply of life-forming organic materials from its own parent interstellar cloud of gas and grains. It did not prove at all difficult to see how such materials could have been acquired by the solar system without suffering disruption by the early heat of the primeval Sun. The materials were simply swept up from the parent cloud, not directly on to the Earth itself, but into the cool distant outermost regions of the solar system, the regions occupied at present by the planets Uranus and Neptune. At that time, however, Uranus and Neptune had not yet formed; their material was divided up among a vast swarm of much smaller bodies to the present-day comets.

We had long believed that the waters of the Earth and the gases of our atmosphere were not original to the Earth, but had been brought here from the outermost regions of the solar system by these same comet-type bodies. And now we had to consider that along with the water and the gases of the atmosphere there might have come great quantities of organic life-forming materials; an amount that might well have been as much as ten per cent of all the waters of the oceans. At first sight, this seemed a considerable help to the orthodox theory that life started here on the Earth, since it provided far more source-material for life than could have been generated locally on the Earth. Before accepting this position, however, we felt it necessary to reconsider an old difficulty, which is that organic molecules are quickly destroyed in the presence of free oxygen. This oxygen problem is so important to the whole question of the origin of life that we shall now consider it at some length.

Imagine the Earth with its present oceans and atmosphere but without life. The higher ground on the land would be mostly bare rock and snow fields. There would be storms as we experience them now. Winds would blow, rain would fall, rivers would flow along courses not significantly different from their present courses. There would be weathering of rocks by wind and water, and sediments would continue to accumulate in river valleys, the beds of lakes, and on the shelves of the continents. But the sediments in the river valleys would not become soil as we understand it, because no organic humus would be added to it from year to year. The world would have a nightmarish topographical similarity to the present Earth. There would be Africa and Asia, Europe and the Americas, but no life to soften the sharp outlines of the landscape. In such a situation could we expect life to begin? The answer is that we could certainly not. The atmosphere and the oceans are made up of very stable inorganic molecules, mostly nitrogen, oxygen, carbon dioxide and water, which do not form themselves into the organic molecules needed for life. Indeed just the opposite. Even if the organic molecules needed for life should be formed in some way they would soon be degraded into simple stable inorganic molecules.

If the life which actually exists on the Earth were all suddenly to die, a very great deal of organic material would at first be left lying around. Yet even such a great quantity of organic material, much of it in the form of complex biomolecules, would not regenerate any life. The material would become degraded into simple inorganic molecules, much of it in a few months. Tree trunk would lie around for some years, and peat bogs in high geographical latitudes would persist for some centuries. But in a time exceedingly short compared to a geological epoch the whole of even such a large initial supply of organic material would be gone.

Oxygen in the atmosphere would be the primary cause of this rapid degradation. Suppose we seek to stop the destructive effect of the oxygen by first adding hydrogen to the atmosphere. The oxygen would then be removed in combination with the hydrogen as water, which would wash out as rain to augment the oceans a little. With this precaution, what would happen if all life were again considered to die suddenly?

In our view the following sequence of events would take place. Any excess of hydrogen that might have been added to the atmosphere would evaporate in a time scale of a few thousand years away into space. The uppermost regions of the atmosphere are surprisingly hot (around the times when sunspots are most numerous in their cycle of about eleven years), and it is this high temperature of about 2000°K that would cause the hydrogen to evaporate and to be lost from the Earth. The high temperature is generated by the absorption during daytime of hard ultraviolet light from the Sun.

While the hydrogen was thus evaporating, softer ultraviolet light from the Sun would penetrate through the Earth's atmosphere to ground level. In particular, ultraviolet that is normally absorbed by ozone (O_2) at a height of twenty-five to fifty kilometres above ground level would come through to the lower atmosphere, where some of it would dissociate water vapour into oxygen and hydrogen. For the several thousand years while hydrogen remained, the oxygen produced in this way would simply recombine with hydrogen back into water. After the hydrogen was gone, however, and with the hydrogen coming from the dissociation of water vapour also escaping into space, oxygen would begin to accumulate. To this point, the reservoir of organic materials would not on the whole have been much degraded. But now, with oxygen accumulating, the reservoir of organic material would again disappear, and we should reach the same final inert situation as before.

The critic will look for a loophole in this argument. Might not the organic materials have regenerated life during the few thousand years in which there was protection by the hydrogen? Our own answer to this question is no. Biologists, however, speak with a forked tongue on the matter. If they are reminded first of Pasteur's destruction of the ancient theory of the spontaneous generation of life, they too will emphatically answer no. Yet, if they are asked the same question in the context of the origin of life 4000 million years ago they will answer yes, and they will do so in circumstances far less favourable than the situation we postulated above. It is therefore ironical that Pasteur, after describing a particularly crucial experiment to the French Academy of Sciences, remarked: 'The theory of spontaneous generation will never recover from this mortal blow.' We provided complex molecules like chlorophyll, cellulose, and even the nucleic acids and proteins in the dead cell of plants and animals. For a proper understanding of the origin of life, the difficult problem of how these complex biomolecules were formed from very much simpler organic molecules must also be solved. Furthermore, we provided a vast quantity of organic material as a starting point.

How, one might ask, do biologists usually suppose that organic molecules were produced? By the effects of ultraviolet light and of lightning strokes in thunderstorms acting on simple inorganic molecules — water, carbon dioxide, methane, amnionia, hydrogen cyanide. These processes break up the simple organic molecules into atoms and radicals which overwhelmingly recombine back into the same simple stable inorganic molecules as before. Only a trickle of the atoms goes into less stable organic molecules. The resulting minuscule organic production on the primitive Earth would fall on to a land surface bare of vegetation, to run off quickly into rivers and thence to the sea, giving rise to no more than trifling concentrations of elementary organic molecules.

We think there is little prospect of combating the above argument by claiming that an early protective hydrogen atmosphere persisted for ten million years or more, rather than for ten thousand years. Astronomical evidence shows that stars are more active at their surfaces when they are young than when they are middle-aged like the Sun. On astronomical grounds we should therefore expect a greater emission of hard ultraviolet light from the young Sun than the Sun emits at present, with the consequence that the protective influence of a hydrogen atmosphere would be shorter than ten thousand years. And in an issue that is really one of deep principle, it is to be doubted that the time scale, so long as it was not obviously too short, is of any relevance at all.

Faced with this problem, it has been customary to take refuge in the assumption that ozone would form from the oxygen. An ozone layer in the high atmosphere, such as the Earth possesses at present, would absorb the damaging ultraviolet light from the Sun, thereby protecting all the water molecules lying below it. The trouble with this idea, however, is that neither oxygen nor ozone could persist in close association with easily burnable organic materials (or mixed with a combustable gas like methane, which is often taken to have been present in the Earth's early atmosphere). So not until after the life-forming materials had been destroyed could ozone begin to accumulate.

How is it then, the reader might wonder, that present-day life manages to coexist with a present-day atmosphere that contains free oxygen? Why does the oxygen not burn up the life? The answer is that it does, very quickly! But life also regenerates itself very quickly, as we emphasised above. Life is perpetually a race against being burned-up by the oxygen, a race that is balanced on a razor's edge and depends crucially on rainfall. When there is plenty of rain, life wins; the environment is everywhere green with grass and trees. When, however, there is only a little rain, burning-up wins, and the landscape is everywhere brown — we have the deserts of the Earth. But of course before there was any life capable of regenerating itself quickly there could have been no such race. In the presence of oxygen, burning-up would win in a canter.

If one had certain knowledge that life really had its beginning here on Earth it would of course be possible to infer an error in the seemingly persuasive argument of the previous paragraphs. The only way to arrive at such knowledge, we reasoned, would be to prove that life could not have begun anywhere else than on the Earth. So we set about seeking such a proof. But instead of arriving at a proof that life could not originate except on the Earth, we found that conditions in comets seemed much better, better particularly in that the oxygen difficulty did not arise at all for comets. So instead of the Earth being merely showered with life-forming materials by comets, we had now to contemplate the idea that the Earth might have been showered by life itself, by a profusion of living cells, some of which had managed to take root here.

If life began on the Earth some four billion years ago, there is not much to be predicted that we do not know already. But if life originated in comets, life must still be there, because the physical conditions in comets are very suitable to its preservation over vast intervals of time. And comets are still with us today — about ten of them come to the vicinity of the Earth each year. So if comets in the distant past shed life on to the Earth, we had to consider the possibility that comets were still doing so today. Suddenly therefore the ideas and theories about the origins of life, apparently rooted in the remote past, sprang for us into the immediate present. Was life in the form of primitive bacteria still reaching the Earth? And could viruses even be derived from comets? The idea seemed preposterous, but in science, one must steel oneself not to decide the correctness or otherwise of ideas according to subjective prejudices. In science, fact reigns supreme. So what were the facts?

Our readings of medical history soon showed examples of diseases that fitted well with the infall on to the Earth of pathogenic viruses and bacteria from space, to a degree where we became convinced that the idea had to be taken quite seriously. We shall review this evidence in later chapters, for the common cold in Chapter 3, for influenza in Chapters 4, 5, 6, and for diseases more generally in Chapter 8. Indeed we found many situations, of which the famous historical incident described at the end of Chapter 2 is an example, where bacteria and viruses from space seemed the only explanation of the facts.

So it came about that the more we read and the more we probed many and diverse arguments, the more surely we were pressed to the strange conclusion that it was in comets where we must seek for the early development of life. Let us return therefore to the addition of organic materials to the outermost regions of the solar system, addition from the particular interstellar cloud within which our solar system was born nearly 5000 million years ago.

In the outer regions of the solar system there was already a vast swarm of hundreds of billions of comet-type bodies. The bodies were hard-frozen mixtures of simple substances, ordinary water, hydrogen cyanide, methane, hydrogen sulphide, to name a few of the commoner ones. It was on top of such hard-frozen mixtures that the interstellar organic materials were deposited. Typically, a cometary body would acquire an organic mantle about a kilometre thick. The organic mantles would initially be hard-frozen like the ices below them, giving conditions that were unsuited to the origin of life. Internal heating and liquefication inevitably occurred, however, as a result of chemical reactions among the organic materials, triggered perhaps by collisions of the comets with smaller bodies. Such reactions could release up to ten times the energy needed to melt cometary ices at a depth of a few hundred metres below the cometary surface, close to the inner boundary with the icy nucleus. High concentrations of organic materials in water solution, along with important inorganics like hydrogen cyanide, would then be maintained for millions of years, because the rate of escape of heat to outside space can be shown to be very slow from regions buried some hundreds of metres below the surface of the cometary objects.

The situation then would be reminiscent of Charles Darwin's idea of a 'warm little pond': '... if (and oh what a big if) we could conceive in some warm little pond, with all sorts of ammonia and phosphoric salts present, that a protein compound was chemically formed ready to undergo still more complex changes ...' The difference is that instead of just one warm little pond, we now might have warm little ponds for thousands of millions of the cometary bodies, ponds which remained warm, not for a few months only, but for millions of years. A further difference is that instead of being supplied with ammonia and phosphoric salts, our ponds are supplied with highly complex organics, perhaps with all the biomolecules that we discussed in our earlier book *Lifecloud* — polysaccharides as an energy source, sugar-phosphate chains and nucleotide bases for the building of proteins, porphyrins for assembly into chlorophyll. Yet another difference is that instead of being exposed to the damaging effect of oxygen in the Earth's atmosphere, our ponds are each safely buried below a kilometre-thick protective skin.

In Appendix 1 we have summarised the astronomical evidence that supports the view that comets are repositories of viral and bacterial life throughout the galaxy. Comets are the first solid bodies to condense during the formation of a new planetary system. They effectively collect bacteria and viruses that exist throughout interstellar space, and amplify a surviving fraction of bacterial cells within their radioactively heated interiors. Since the first direct observations of comets were made following the advent of the space age, beginning with the studies of the nucleus of comet Halley in 1986, evidence for comets carrying bacteria and viruses has grown to the point of being overwhelming. The most recent data from the Rosetta mission to comet 67P/C-G yielded wealth of data supporting such a picture.

While the majority of the comet-type objects we have been discussing went to form the planets Uranus and Neptune, a fraction must have been sprayed inwards to the central regions of the solar system, and a fraction was very likely sprayed outwards to form the giant halo around the solar system that we identify as the present-day comets. An inwardly deflected comet on which biological evolution had occurred could have seeded our planet with life some 4000 million years ago. The seeding could have occurred in a large-scale cometary landing, or it could have occurred more gradually through accumulations of cometary material that became dispersed into fine micrometeoritic particles. With each passage of a comet past the Sun, the outer layers are gradually peeled away, the process continuing until the one-time biochemically active ponds, now re-frozen, are eventually exposed at the surface. The freezing would ensure the preservation of cometary viruses and bacteria for almost indefinite periods. It is the eventual evaporation of such frozen surfaces that leads to the formation of the visible and famous 'tails' of comets, and also to the broadcasting of particles, some of which in our view contain viruses and some of which are bacteria.

Bacteria evolving within comets are of necessity anaerobic, i.e. out of contact with free oxygen. A small fraction of cometary bacteria which enter the Earth's atmosphere could conceivably make a transition from the anaerobic state to an aerobic one, although the vast majority may have perished. Aerobic bacteria on the Earth may have originated in this way, namely as the surviving members of the astronomically large number of cells which were shed from comets. Viruses could be carried within living cells, or they could be encapsulated in particles of either organic or inorganic composition.

From the arguments presented in this first chapter we find that the case for a cometary origin of life, as well as for a continuing infall on to the Earth of bacteria and viruses, is reasonably established on a preliminary basis. Accepting this position, at first tentatively, we shall proceed in succeeding chapters to discuss evidence and arguments that transform what at first seems an implausible hypothesis to a position with strong factual support.

2
Pathogenic Invaders

The journey for a bacterium or virus from the interior of a comet to the surface of the Earth is fraught with considerable hazard, and it is likely that only a small fraction of all bacteria and viruses would make the transfer safely. But because of its penchant for huge numbers, biology is well-geared to situations in which many perish, so long as the few survive.

If it were not for the terrestrial atmosphere, safe arrival at the Earth's surface would not be possible at all. Incoming small particles would impact the hard ground directly, and would be instantly gasified, as they must be on striking the Moon. This is the reason why space-incident bacteria and viruses cannot be found at the surface of the Moon. Yet while the Earth's atmosphere provides for a comparatively 'soft' landing, it does not remove all hazards. Entry at high speed of a particle into the atmosphere inevitably produces a heating of the particle. The smaller the particle, however, the cooler it remains as it is slowed from its initially high speed by the Earth's upper atmosphere (the slowing down occurs at a height of about 120 kilometres above ground level).

The sizes of bacteria and viruses are therefore very relevant to pathogens remaining cool enough not to become 'sterilised', and in this connection the sizes of bacteria and of some well-known viruses illustrated in Figure 2.2 are important. The calculations we give in Appendix 2 show that for the size scale of viruses there is no possibility of a space pathogen becoming 'cooked'. Destruction through atmospheric heating usually comes when the size scale is around 1μ. (The reader is reminded that 1μ, known as the micron, is one-millionth of a metre. The *nanometre,* nm, is one-thousandth of a *micron,* so that the left-hand scale of Figure 2.2 is *one tenth* of the right-hand scale.) Except in the special case discussed in Appendix 2, we find that to exceed about 1μ, a bacterium must be rod-shaped (since it is the diameter of the rod rather than its length which matters critically in the heating problem), as indeed the large bacteria in Figure 2.2 can be seen to be. The dimensions of some common bacteria, given more precisely in Table 2.1, fit the heating requirement exceedingly well. According to our theory, bacteria are just about as big as they can possibly be.

The infall from space of a particular pathogen would necessarily be an irregular process, intermittent in time because of its position

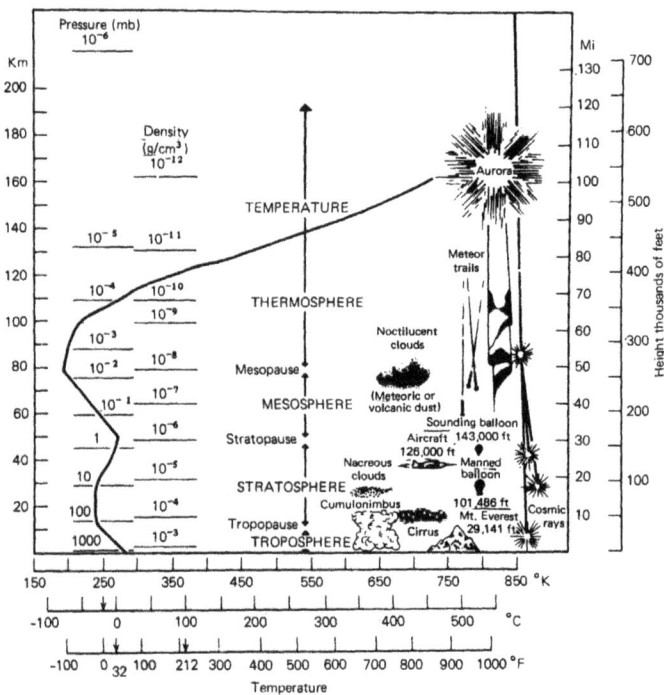

Fig. 2.1.   Schematic representation of the temperature and density profiles of the atmosphere, showing divisions into a thermosphere, mesosphere, stratosphere and troposphere. Also shown are the heights attained by balloon and rocket flights, and by various cloud formations.

Table 2.1.   The shapes and sizes of some bacteria.

---

(1) *Cocci*
Straphylococci
Streptococci   Each cell is approximately a sphere with radius 0.5μ
Pneumococci

---

(2) *Bacilli (rods)*

Mycobacterium Tuberculosis:	0.3μ diameter, 3μ length
Escherichia Coli:	0.5μ diameter, $3-5\mu$ length
Clostridium Tetani:	0.5μ diameter, 5μ length
Pasteurellae Pestis:	0.7μ diameter, 1.5μ length
Brucellae Abortus:	0.4μ diameter, 0.6μ length

---

(3) *Vibrios (wavy shape)*

Vibrio Cholerae:	0.5μ diameter, $2-3\mu$ length

---

and motion relative to the Earth, and patchy in its incidence on the Earth's surface because of meteorological factors. If the source in space is a sharply defined volume (as in a different connection the shadow cast by the Moon is sharply defined) then the pathogen will be limited in its incidence to a particular area of the Earth's surface, like the particular area to which one must go to witness an eclipse of the Sun. On the other hand, the pathogen may have a much wider spatial distribution, in which case it will be incident over the whole Earth. Yet the moment of first arrival at ground level of a widely distributed pathogen may vary between the different continents of the Earth by weeks, months or even years. This is because small particles fall only slowly down through the upper atmosphere. The structure and temperature distribution of the atmosphere, with its divisions into a thermosphere, mesosphere, stratosphere, and troposphere, are shown schematically in Figure 2.1. Particles with diameters of a hundredth of a millimetre (from our point of view these would be quite large) fall under their individual motions down through the stratosphere in two or three months. Particles much smaller than this do not fall individually, however, but are carried along by the general air movements of the upper air, or are dragged downwards by electrical forces (for a discussion of the latter, see L. C. Hale, *Nature,* Vol 268, 710, 1977).

Once below the base of the stratosphere (which occurs at a height above ground level of about fifteen kilometres over the tropics and at about ten kilometres over the temperate zones) particles are carried down to the lower atmosphere in rain or snow in a matter of days or weeks. Small particles may, however, remain in the stratosphere for time-scales of the order five to ten years. This is known from the persistence there of fine dust thrown up high in the violent explosions of volcanoes.

The critical features in the descent of small particles (micro-meteorites) from space is the transition from the stratosphere to the troposphere, and it is this transition that is highly variable from one location on the Earth to another. For particles of the size scale of viruses, the electrical forces may arise from very large terrestrial thunderstorms, or they may be space incident, as for instance from storms on the Sun which cause disturbances in the so-called auroral belt of the earth.

For particles on the size scale of bacteria (see Figure 2.2) violent storms in the lower atmosphere can set up eddy exchanges with the air in the stratosphere, and so storms could bring a pathogen down to ground level. Interchange also occurs from air currents moving around the tracks of the two jet streams which circle the Earth, one in each geographical hemisphere. Thus the track of each jet stream, typically in latitude 30° in winter and in latitude 45° in summer, is also a region of breakthrough between the stratosphere and the troposphere.

Let us suppose that atmospheric eddies produce a patchy situation, shown schematically in Figure 2.3, in which the dark areas are the regions of fall of a disease-causing virus or bacterium. For a human disease, a person living a sedentary life may be engulfed by one of the dark spots of Figure 2.3, or alternatively the place of residence may lie in a vacant area of the figure. There is a chance of making contact with the disease and a chance of avoiding it, the chances being determined by the fraction of the ground area

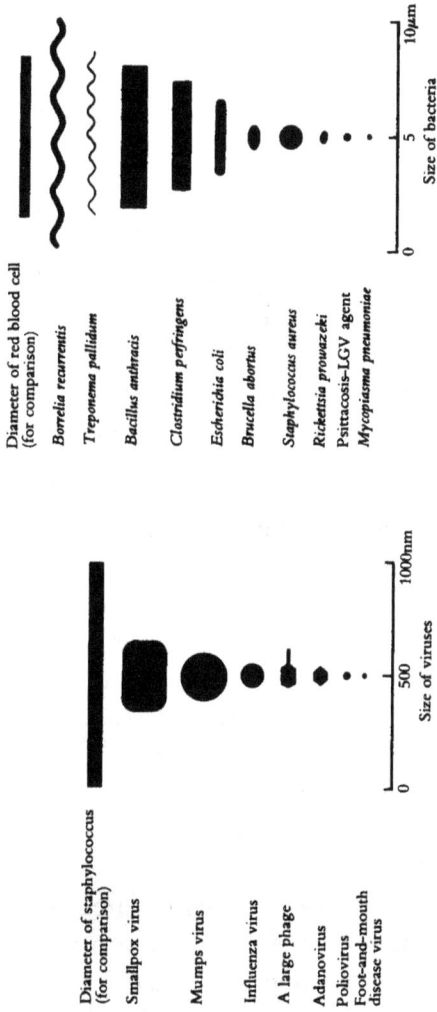

Diameter of red blood cell
(for comparison)
Borrelia recurrentis
Treponema pallidum
Bacillus anthracis
Clostridium perfringens
Escherichia coli
Brucella abortus
Staphylococcus aureus
Rickettsia prowazeki
Psittacosis-LGV agent
Mycoplasma pneumoniae

Size of bacteria

Diameter of staphylococcus
(for comparison)
Smallpox virus
Mumps virus
Influenza virus
A large phage
Adanovirus
Poliovirus
Foot-and-mouth
disease virus

Size of viruses

Fig. 2.2. Sizes and shapes of bacteria and viruses: $1\mu m = 1$ millionth and $1nm = 1000$ millionth of a metre (adapted from C. G. A. Thomas, *Medical Microbiology*, London, 1973).

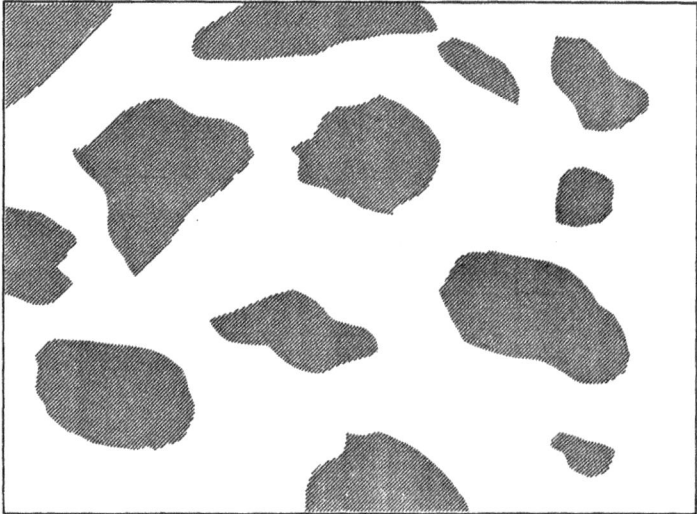

Fig. 2.3. Schematic representation of pathogenic clouds settling at ground level. The patches (shaded areas) cover about one third of the total surface.

covered by the dark blobs of Figure 2.3. The persistent traveller, however, even if fortunate to be initially in a clear area, will sooner or later move into one or other of the pathogenic patches. Travellers — seamen, for example — are therefore more vulnerable to catching diseases than, say, farmers. In the days before air travel, when boat journeys with long periods at sea were frequent, there were often reports of epidemics occurring many days after leaving the last port of call. After recovering, passengers would sometimes to their astonishment find the disease had already arrived ahead of them at the next port of call.

Where a pathogen falls over an entire area, Figure 2.3 is still likely to be representative of the situation at a particular moment, but with the detailed positioning of the dark blobs then changing with time. In this more extreme case, all who are in the area, traveller and sedentary person alike, are eventually hit by the bacterium or virus. The difference now is that, whereas the traveller is almost always hit early, the sedentary person may be hit either early or late, more likely not early if the dark patches at any one moment form only a modest fraction of the total area. This relation of pattern-to-movement explains a situation we shall encounter in Chapters 3 and 4, in which moving boats in the neighbourhood of an island are hit a little ahead in time of the island itself. When in such a situation a stricken boat happens to call at the island, the illusion of the boat having 'brought' the disease to the island is created, an illusion with a simple explanation in terms of Figure 2.3.

Among the animals, far-flying birds are particularly exposed to attack, since they are inevitably going to move sooner or later into one or more of the dark blobs of Figure 2.3. Hence we may expect birds to have evolved better immunities than more or less sedentary land animals have done. For influenza, the most carefully studied cross-species disease, this is certainly so.

The patches of Figure 2.3 can be generated at ground-level by local obstacles — hills, woodland areas, buildings — as well as by natural eddies of the air. As another example, hot air near a furnace must tend to destroy pathogens, thus producing a clear area in the figure. A very fine scale patchiness is therefore to be expected, especially over heavily populated urban areas.

An incoming virus or bacterium my or may not be attacking; there are many non-pathogenic varieties of bacteria that simply lie around in the soil, indefinitely if not destroyed by water or by the temperature of their surroundings. Even the attacking varieties could fail in some cases to interact with terrestrial life forms, through being washed into rivers and thence into the sea. But where attack occurs, the bacterium or virus in question succeeds in establishing for itself a reservoir that grows through multiplication of the pathogen in the host plant or animal.

The reservoir which an attacking virus or bacterium succeeds in establishing for itself may be evanescent or it may be long-lived. The influenza virus in humans has not been found to persist for more than a few weeks, whereas the reservoir of the influenza virus in birds is longer–lived. Before the advent of modern health procedures, the smallpox reservoir persisted in humans on a time-scale certainly of many years and probably of some centuries.

The reservoir of the virus *herpes simplex,* which causes cold sores on the lips, is persistent on a still longer time-scale, probably of many thousands of years. Yet in our view, every pathogenic reservoir eventually dies away if it is not renewed from outside, in a time interval much shorter than the times required for major evolutionary changes among the higher animals. We would argue that ten thousand years ago there were no reservoirs for most of the infectious diseases that afflict mankind today.

It is a consequence of these ideas that the aim of ridding the world of all infectious diseases is another illusion. Many medical authorities believe that the World Health Organisation (WHO) has finally rid the world of smallpox. But the world has been rid of smallpox before. As we shall see in Chapter 8, smallpox seems to have been rife in Egypt in the days of Moses, but it was apparently unknown to classical Greece and Rome. The likelihood is that smallpox will return one day to the Earth, though it is to be hoped that this will not happen until very many centuries from now. Other diseases of which we have no present knowledge will also arrive in the future.

It is a further consequence of these ideas that in the past there must have been diseases of which we have no present knowledge. An astonishingly virulent and remarkably localised disease struck the city of Athens in the summer of 430 BC. The symptoms of the disease are so unlike anything known to modern medicine that some authorities have wondered if the account of it by Thucydides in *The Peloponnesian Wars* could possibly be in error, and it might perhaps seem curious that the description comes to us from the 'father of history', rather than from Hippocrates the 'father of medicine'. The details of the life of Hippocrates are scanty, however, and it seems likely that the name survives as a tradition rather than as a person.

Because of the importance of what Thucydides had to say, because it strikes at the very heart of our ideas on the origins of infectious disease, it is worth pausing to take a brief look at the life and character of Thucydides himself. When the first Peloponnesian War broke out in 431 BC Thucydides set himself to keep a personal diary. As the conflict continued down the years (it ended twentyseven years later in 404 BC) Thucydides broadened his aim to include in his history every significant battle and every relevant political manoeuvre that took place, not just between Athens and Sparta, but among the many Greek cities involved in the fighting. The mounting complexity, combined with a compulsion for total accuracy, ultimately caused Thucydides to stop writing in 411 BC. Ageing himself, surrounded as we may imagine by a multitude of disconnected notes, he came to put off the task of finally organising his material, exactly as so many scholars have done in later ages. As P. A. Brunt says in the Introduction to *The Great Histories* series under the editorship of Hugh Trevor-Roper: 'Perhaps his passion for accuracy and the difficulty he had in ascertaining the exact truth every time delayed him as he wrote and rewrote in quest of perfection.'

So let us come to what Thucydides actually had to say of the Plague of Athens. The writing has tremendous momentum and a needle-sharp clarity that contrasts favourably with most writings, both modern and ancient.

The season was universally admitted to have been remarkably free from other sicknesses; and if anybody was already ill of any other disease, it finally turned into this. The other victims who were in perfect health, all in a moment and without any exciting cause, were seized first with violent heats in the head and with redness and burning of the eyes. Internally, the throat and the tongue at once became blood-red, and the breath abnormal and fetid. Sneezing and hoarseness followed; in a short time the disorder, accompanied by a violent cough, reached the chest. And whenever it settled in the heart, it upset it; and there were all the vomits of bile to which physicians have ever given names, and they were accompanied by great distress. An ineffectual retching, producing violent convulsions, attacked most of the sufferers; some, as soon as the previous symptoms had abated, others, not until long afterwards. The body externally was not so very hot to the touch, not yellowish but flushed and livid and breaking out in blisters and ulcers. But the internal fever was intense; the sufferers could not bear to have on them even the lightest linen garments; they insisted on being naked, and there was nothing which they longed for more eagerly than to throw themselves into cold water, many of those who had no one to look after them actually plunged into the cisterns. They were tormented by unceasing thirst, which was not in the least assuaged whether they drank much or little. They could find no way of resting, and sleeplessness attacked them throughout. While the disease was at its height, the body, instead of wasting away, held out amid these sufferings unexpectedly. Thus, most died on the seventh to ninth day of internal fever, though their strength was not exhausted; or, if they survived, then the disease descended into the bowels and there produced violent lesions; at the same time diarrhoea set in which was uniformly fluid, and at a later stage caused exhaustion, and this finally carried them off with few exceptions. For the disorder which had originally settled in the head passed gradually through the whole body and, if a person got over the worst, would often seize the extremities and leave its mark, attacking the privy parts, fingers and toes; and many escaped with the loss of these, some with the loss of their eyes. Some again had no sooner recovered than they were seized with a total loss of memory and knew neither themselves nor their friends.

The character of the malady no words can describe, and the fury with which it fastened upon each sufferer was too much for human nature to endure. There was one circumstance in particular which distinguished it from ordinary diseases. Although so many bodies were lying unburied, the birds and animals which feed on human flesh either never came near them or died if they touched them. This is the evidence: there was a manifest disappearance of birds of prey, which were not to be seen either near the bodies or anywhere else; while in the case of the dogs what happened was even more obvious because they live with man.

Attempts to cover all the symptoms described here by Thucydides in terms of modern diseases have failed. To some, the breaking out in blisters and ulcers has suggested smallpox. To others, the thirst and the impulse of the victims to throw themselves into the 'cisterns' has suggested cholera. Yet how, even if one combined both of these diseases, does one explain the 'loss' of the eyes, toes and fingers? 'Loss' presumably means blindness in the case of the eyes, and paralysis in the case of fingers and toes. To still others, the 'internal fever' that caused sufferers to insist on lying naked has even suggested ergot, a far-fetched notion indeed. The consensus of opinion, however, is that if the description of Thucydides is correct the plague of Athens was a disease quite unknown to modern medical science. Yet to suggest that Thucydides, a man with a complete mastery of words, a man who observed the disease at first hand over an extended period, who took the greatest pains to use precise medical terms throughout his description, was in gross error, surely borders on the ridiculous. So here was a deadly disease, unknown before and unknown since. Where did it come from and where did it go? Here is one problem among many for those who prefer the conventional theory of infectious diseases to the theory we discuss in this book.

3

The Viral Connection

We remarked in Chapter 2 that a successful attack on a terrestrial plant or animal establishes a reservoir for an invading pathogen. The reservoir may have long-term persistence, or it may be short-lived, depending on the survival characteristics of the particular bacterium or virus. Once they are exposed in naked form (i.e. without a surrounding protective matrix such as viruses and bacteria from space would need to have), the viruses of the common cold and of influenza quickly lose their ability to attack the respiratory tracts of their hosts. The smallpox virus, on the other hand, is able to persist in a free form for many years outside of any human, and can therefore remain lying around for an extended period waiting to renew its assault. Such persistence gives the smallpox virus an important advantage in maintaining itself, compared to the viruses of influenza and the common cold. Indeed, the latter cannot maintain themselves at all as reservoirs except through continuing incorporation within their hosts. Continuing presence within the host is by no means an unknown phenomenon — the herpes virus persists readily within humans. Neither influenza nor the common cold, however, has been shown to persist within humans, although influenza virus has been found in birds, and in certain other animal (cf. Table 4.2).

It has therefore seemed attractive to those who favour the orthodox theory of infectious diseases to suppose that the reservoir of the influenza virus lies within animals other than ourselves. The immediate difficulty with this point of view is that the influenza virus exists in several types, each with many subtypes, and that the subtypes which are found in other animals are not in themselves of the right kind to attack humans in a clearly infectious way. Our view is that influenza is found in both humans and animals because we are all subject to the incidence of pathogens from space, with the different types and subtypes of influenza virus picking out the particular terrestrial species that they are best able to attack. According to our point of view, pathogens like influenza and the common cold, which are the ones without detectable human reservoirs, must be renewed frequently and almost continuously from space, otherwise they would quickly become extinct. Hence in looking for evidence of the incidence of diseases from space, it is to continuously driven cases like influenza and the common cold that we naturally turn, rather than to potentially long-persisting diseases like smallpox. The reason, of course, is that the incidence of smallpox from space, if it occurred many centuries ago, would not be susceptible to present-day investigation.

In this chapter we shall discuss the common cold, and in several following chapters we shall be concerned with the strange epidemiology of influenza. In particular, we shall be interested in the question of whether or not these diseases are passed at all readily from one person to another, for if person-to-person transmission can be shown not to take place then it becomes hard to avoid the conclusion that viruses do indeed settle down on to us from the atmosphere.

At first sight, one might think the only procedure for verifying the cometary theory of the origin of life would be directly through a space voyage to an actual comet, by acquiring material there and by returning to Earth with it. While we believe that visiting a comet would inevitably have great scientific interest, we ourselves have no explicit practical part to play in deciding whether or not such a space voyage will be made in the future. We have therefore turned our thoughts in other directions. We thought of high-flying aircraft collecting micrometeorites from space, using a technique essentially similar to the catching of flies with sticky paper. The sticky paper would be returned to Earth, the microparticles picked off it individually, and then examined for their inner contents. In principle, one could then check to see if reproductive viruses and bacteria were present. But since many hundreds, and perhaps thousands, of tons of material in the form of micrometeorites enter the Earth's atmosphere each year, this procedure could prove exceedingly laborious. If as little as one part in a hundred million of this material were influenza virus, the amount of virus would be sufficient to generate a worldwide pandemic. One might therefore need access to a very large number of micrometeorites before finding a single virus-containing particle.

Our next idea was to examine ice-cores taken from Greenland or from the Antarctic, since micrometeorites fall there in snow storms and then become hard-frozen for many thousands of years within the glaciers. Upon thawing, many of the bacteria and viruses within the micrometeorites would be still viable even after great intervals of time. We think this would be the least expensive way to acquire material from space, although there is the clear disadvantage for bacteria that the problem would arise of distinguishing extraterrestrial bacteria from those of terrestrial origin that have arrived in the polar regions through being lifted into the air and blown there by winds from lower latitudes. And for viruses there is the further practical difficulty that techniques for separating a tiny quantity of virus from a vast mass of ice do not at present exist. This, it may be noted, explains why it would be hopeless to seek to prove or disprove the idea of bacteria and viruses from comets by spacecraft sent to Mars, at any rate by present-day spacecraft. The experiments that can be performed at the surface of Mars are necessarily crude compared to what could be done in the Arctic regions of the Earth; and if the latter are at the moment inadequate, so quite evidently are the former.

Although these thoughts turned out to be rather disappointingly negative, there is fortunately a positive side to the situation. Much the most sensitive detectors of virus are plants and animals themselves. It needs only a few influenza virus particles deposited in the throat to send a person down with this potentially lethal disease. No laboratory detector could compare with the explosive response of a person to the virus. Therefore the medical facts concerning actual diseases give the most delicate information concerning the incidence of a pathogen from space. The complicating issues are those we have discussed already, the establishment of pathogenic reservoirs, and the infection of one plant or animal by another. Yet if the facts indicate an absence of contagion, as we ourselves think they do for influenza, and perhaps also for the common cold, and furthermore if the virus in question has no known reservoir, the complications do not arise. The problem then simplifies to one of incidence only. It is for this reason that we shall be so concerned in this and succeeding chapters with the issue of person-to-person transmission. While the existence of this lateral type of transmission of a disease does not contradict the idea of a cometary origin of viruses and bacteria, the absence of person-to-person transmission, particularly for respiratory diseases, would go a long way towards proving the idea.

Either way, person-to-person transmission or incidence from space, we must expect two persons associating together often both to come down with a cold or with influenza. There will be an important difference, however, in the timing of the onset of clinical symptoms. Thus if two persons associating together are hit by the same pathogenic patch (Figure 2.3) both victims will come down with the disease more or less contemporaneously. But for an infection passed from one person to another, clinical symptoms will be separated in time by approximately the incubation period of the disease.

To fix ideas, it will be useful to have a few numbers in mind. Clinical symptoms generally show themselves when the number of virus particles per cubic centimetre of infected tissue is about 10,000 million. It follows that for diseases like the cold and influenza, diseases that can explode from a single virus particle in some two to three days, the doubling time for the virus must on the average be about two hours. It also follows that for a high initial infection, say ten thousand virus particles per cubic centimetre, clinical symptoms will follow in only about a day and a half. However, under natural conditions — for instance, in schools or public gatherings — such high initial infections must be rare (if infections occur at all) since for doses as high as ten thousand virus particles per cubic centimetre, it would be essentially impossible for any susceptible person to escape the disease. Yet in most influenza epidemics, and in most waves of the common cold, the majority of susceptible people do in fact escape, which implies that most doses must be marginal — i.e. just a few virus particles or none. Hence we can say that under natural conditions the incubation periods of influenza and of the common cold must usually be some two to three days. Along a chain of person-to-person transmission it would therefore take a time of about two and a half days to pass from one link of the chain to the next. From a single case of influenza or of the common cold, it would take about ten days for the disease to spread through a group of, say, fifty persons. By way of contrast to this rather slow spread by person-to-person transmission, we shall find many examples of outbreaks of these diseases that are much swifter in their onset than this.

Before we proceed, there is a further detail concerned with incidence from space. According to our point of view the influenza virus or the common cold virus does not reach a person's throat in a free form. It would either be encased in a protective matrix of some kind — an inorganic mineral, an organic capsule consisting perhaps of cellulose — or even contained within an accompanying bacterium. Not until a virus could free itself from the surrounding matrix would infection occur. In some cases, incident microparticles would be coughed away, or washed down into the stomach, a circumstance that in our view explains the seemingly capricious incidence of respiratory diseases. Some people contract colds in a wave, or influenza in an epidemic, while others escape, a difference that could turn on simple points like the drinking of fluid at a particular moment. We should also add the observation that mild gastroenteritis, cases of which often occur with the 'bug' unidentified, could in our view be due to pathogens which in a free form would have remained in the respiratory tract, but which in a protective matrix are able to reach the stomach.

It is estimated that more working days are lost from the common cold than through any other single cause, a melancholy situation that has persisted in human society for a long time, right from the golden age of classical Greece or before, as we can see in the following quotation from Hippocrates:

> In the first place, those of us who suffer from cold in the head, with discharge from the nostrils, generally find this discharge more acrid than that which previously formed there and daily passed from the nostrils; it makes the nose swell, and inflames it to an extremely fiery heat, as is shown if you put your hand upon it. And if the disease be present for an unusually long time, the part actually becomes ulcerated, although it is without flesh and hard. But in some way the heat of the nostril ceases, not when the discharge takes place and the inflammation is present, but when the running becomes thicker and less acrid, being matured and more mixed than it was before, then it is that the heat finally ceases. But in cases where the evil obviously comes from cold alone, unaccompanied by anything else, there is always the same change, heat following chill and chill heat, and these supervene at once, and need no coction ...

Common cold symptoms vary considerably from one individual to another, although in the same individual the same symptoms tend to recur with repeated infections. The symptoms may include sneezing, headache, tiredness, chilling, sore nose, sore throat and nasal discharge. There is usually no appreciable fever, however, and it is this which permits us to 'carry on', albeit with an effort, through most of the phases of a cold. For an adult the average attack is thought to be some two to three colds per year, while young children tend to suffer a higher rate of six to twelve per year. These numbers depend upon what one defines as a 'cold': a so-called 'stinker' or only a minor snuffle? The present estimates are for occasions on which we feel a real measure of inconvenience. Minor snuffles occur at least twice as frequently as do severe colds.

It is the sheer persistence of the attack which gives to the common cold its great nuisance value. In our view, persistence indicates an almost continuous incidence of the virus on to the Earth from space. The Earth is perpetually immersed in a cloud of micrometeorites, some of them always containing the common cold virus. We would also argue that it is the continuing incidence, rather than an incidence in one sudden pulse, which explains why there are so many (perhaps a hundred) varieties of the virus — the Earth simply picks up everything that is going.

The generally innocuous course of the common cold disease makes it difficult to come by accurate epidemiological data for the disease. Memories of past colds soon become vague. Medical authorities only record colds under special circumstances, which can all too readily introduce psychological bias into the data. It is necessary to appraise prospective victims in advance of catching the disease, informing them that they have become a part of some 'experiment'. Unless the experiment is carefully designed to exclude bias, there will inevitably be a falsification of data, a phenomenon well known to astronomers for two centuries or more. As an example, an astronomer might wish to measure precise positions for a number of objects — for instance stars — on a stack of photographic plates. What is done is to shuffle the plates into a random unknown order with unknown orientations, so that the astronomer has no idea of which object he happens at any moment to be measuring. This procedure is known to defeat psychological bias, which shows itself immediately as soon as the astronomer knows ahead of measurement the nature of each object and the potential significance to be attached to each measurement. In like manner, it is desirable for epidemiological data to be collected only from victims who are entirely unaware at the time of suffering a disease that at a subsequent date they are to become the subject of an 'experiment'. When in a later chapter on influenza, we come to discuss epidemiological data that we ourselves have collected, this important criterion will be seen to be satisfied.

The innocuous nature of the common cold unfortunately forces victims to be made aware in advance that they are to be the subject of an investigation. For reliability, conditions similar to a laboratory experiment then become essential, and it is therefore important that already in 1946 the British Medical Council decided to set up a Common Cold Research Unit, based on a former US Army hospital sited a mile and a half to the south-west of Salisbury. Dr D. K. M. Chalmers was responsible for much of the early planning of this

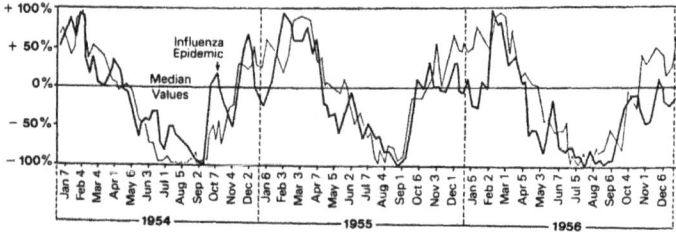

Fig. 3.1. Incidence of the common cold (heavy line) compared with ground temperature (thin line) as a function of time (after R. E. Hope-Simpson).

Unit, and Sir Christopher Andrewes was its first director. Much of what we know with precision about the common cold has come from this far-sighted innovation by the Medical Research Council.

It is interesting to compare epidemiological data with precisely controlled research in the assessment of the age-old prejudice that one catches a cold through being chilled, as for instance through sitting around for some hours in wet clothing. Figure 3.1 gives data obtained by the Gloucestershire physician Dr R. E. Hope-Simpson and shows a remarkable correlation between soil temperatures (one foot below ground surface) and the frequency of incidence of colds among Dr Hope-Simpson's patients. From these data Dr Hope-Simpson drew the conclusion, in our view correctly, that colds arc caused by seasonal effects, not by person-to-person transmission. It would be possible, however, to interpret Figure 3.1 naively by arguing that the data confirmed the old prejudice that people catch cold through being cold. We should therefore consider what a controlled experiment showed. In his book *The Common Cold* Sir Christopher Andrewes writes:

> The belief that cold causes colds is so widespread as, in most people's minds, to admit of no question. In one enquiry 64% of those questioned thought their colds were brought on by chilling. Nevertheless, experimental proof is lacking. Experiments to test the matter were carried out at the Salisbury Unit. In the first

experiment we took three groups with six volunteers in each. These, it may be said, specially volunteered for the rather harsh treatment we gave them. Three pairs took hot baths and thereafter stood about in bathing attire, undried, in a cool corridor for half an hour or as long as they could stand it. Then they were allowed to dress but still wore wet socks for some hours. Most of them had a considerable drop in body temperature and felt rather chilled and miserable. Three other pairs received the dilute virus plus the special chilling treatment. Chilling alone produced no colds. The group receiving virus alone developed two colds; those with chilling and dilute virus got four colds...

Within the uncertainty of the experiment, the implication is that the physical act of chilling or wetting alone, without the virus, has no effect on the incidence of colds. Exposure to the real weather and to real rain, which might be formed around micrometeorites containing the cold virus, could of course be another matter.

If temperature is not in itself the cause of our catching colds, how then are we to interpret Figure 3.1? The data show that colds are most frequent when the ground is coldest, and least frequent when the ground is warmest. During the year, sea temperatures vary by much less than ground temperatures. Hence the temperature difference between sea and land is mainly determined by the heating and cooling of the land surface. When the land is coldest, around February, the temperature difference between the sea and land has its largest positive value, and it is then that a thermodynamic engine carrying heat from sea to land can have its greatest efficiency. Consequently in late winter the greatest rain-bearing storms sweep from the sea on to the land. Such storms produce eddy transfers into the stratosphere and they also generate electrical fields that reach far up into the stratosphere. The direction of these fields is such that they usually pull downwards small micrometeorites which otherwise would take years to fall through still air. To be effective, this process requires the particles to be less than about five millionths of a centimetre in diameter, a condition satisfied by virus particles. Thus small micrometeorites are dragged down through the Earth's upper atmosphere more effectively in winter than they are in summer. A marked seasonal effect for the incidence of small virus-containing micrometeorites is therefore to be expected.

The work of the Salisbury Unit is widely accepted as having demonstrated that colds are not easily transmitted among normal populations. To quote Sir Christopher Andrewes again:

> Eight normal people were exposed for ten hours to inoculated volunteers at a time when the latter, twenty-four to thirty-six hours after inoculation, were still free from symptoms. Eleven others were similarly exposed to people with full-blown colds. The only contact to catch a cold was one who stayed with the pre-symptomatic persons. In fact, in this and in several similar experiments, we noted an extremely low occurrence of successful spread by contact...

How then are we to explain the frequent experience that co-ordinated waves of common cold spread within a week or two over vast tracts of country, as for instance over much of the United States? It has been suggested that the virus may spread at a much slower rate, first in a latent non-symptomatic form, later to be activated more or less simultaneously by some natural event. There are no facts, however, to support such a view. The activation hypothesis is simply an *ad hoc* attempt to avoid the far more cogent inference, namely that waves of the common cold occur because of a nearly simultaneous fall of the virus over widely extended geographical areas.

We turn now from people living in large populations like the UK and the USA to persons living in small isolated communities. The usual view of this problem is that once contact with the outside world is broken, the cold virus dies out within a few months. The people then rapidly lose immunity to the virus and so become exceedingly susceptible to its re-introduction as soon as contact with the outside world is re-established.

The patchy-incidence picture of Figure 2.3 leads to a partially similar situation. Unlike a large community, some parts of which will inevitably be hit by pathogenic patches and other parts of which will escape, a small isolated community will either be hit as a whole or it will escape as a whole. Whereas a large community tends to show an average of Figure 2.3, an isolated community is in an all-or-nothing situation, with an attack-rate either of zero or of essentially a hundred per cent. Just as is the case with the usual view, the possibilities are more extreme for an isolated community than they are for a large geographically extended population.

As well as similarities, however, there are important differences. Our view of the problem is not dependent on any presumption of a markedly varying immunity, which, for a virus with as many varieties as the common cold, we suspect to be a dubious proposition. And our view does not permit an isolated community to escape infection indefinitely, even if the community refrains from re-establishing contact with the outside world. An interesting verification of this expectation has been reported by T. R. Allen, A. F. Bradburne, E. J. Stott, C. S. Goodwin and D. A. J. Tyrrell of the British Antarctic Survey. Of twelve men who had lived seventeen weeks in complete isolation, all but two went down within a week with colds in varying degrees of severity. The authors remark: 'examination of specimens taken from the men in relation to the outbreak has not revealed a causative agent.' Many similarly unexplained outbreaks have been reported from ships at sea.

Data from the island of Tristan da Cunha (37.15S, 12.3W) have been obtained by M. Shibli, S. Gooch, H. E. Lewis and D. A. J. Tyrrell and are shown in Figure 3.2. The experience of the inhabitants of Tristan da Cunha is exactly as we expect, long periods essentially free of colds, punctuated by violent epidemic pulses. It will be seen that boats call in quite frequently at the island, and that in the great majority of cases no epidemic ensues. There are particular cases, however, in which epidemic outbursts appear to follow shortly after the calling of a boat, in September 1964 (although a boat calling a week earlier did not cause colds), in January 1965, in mid-April 1966, and at the end of April 1967. With four out of the eight epidemic outbursts shown in Figure 3.2 thus associated closely in time with boats, some non-random connection is clearly implied. The connection need not,

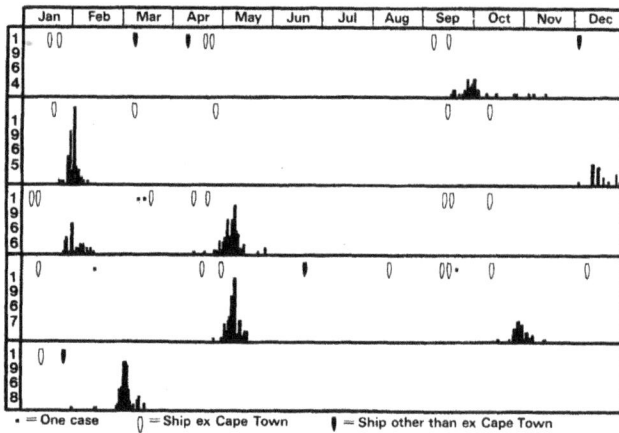

Fig. 3.2. Epidemics of the respiratory disease in Tristan da Cunha (from M. Shibli *et al., Journal of Hygiene,* Cambridge, 69, 255, 1971).

however, be the one suggested by Dr Shibli and his colleagues, namely that the islanders were infected by seamen from the boats. Indeed there appears to us to be compelling evidence against this suggestion. First, it leaves the other four epidemic outbursts unexplained. Second, the islanders spent 1962 and 1963 in England, following a volcanic eruption on Tristan da Cunha in 1961, and so they would have returned home with a more or less normal immunity to the common cold virus. Third, the boats call at the island often enough to prevent immunity falling low.

We pointed out in Chapter 2 that boats are particularly likely to encounter one or other of the pathogenic patches of Figure 2.3, so that if a boat is not initially in a patch, it moves around until it eventually arrives in one. It follows on a statistical basis that boats in the vicinity of Tristan da Cunha were more likely to be hit than the island itself. Hence in those cases where the island happened to be hit, it is quite likely that one or more boats in the vicinity would also be hit probably ahead in time. The boats, being mostly engaged in fishing, called at Tristan da Cunha from time to time for supplies, presumably on no particular fixed schedules. We suspect that when a boat was smitten with colds, with the men feeling physically lethargic, a decision would sometimes have been made to put in at the island and so make 'use' of the few days during which the crew members were below par. If so, the four correlations of Figure 3.2 are psychological in origin, a possibility that always arises when situations are not under planned control.

An interesting planned experiment, however, was carried out by the Salisbury Unit. Again to quote Sir Christopher Andrewes:

We planned therefore to keep the whole thing under our own control by marooning our own party of explorers on our own desert island. We learnt through Dr Fraser Darling of a suitable island, Eilean nan Ron, lying one and half miles off the little port of Skerray on the north coast of Sutherland. It was just over a mile long and less than a mile wide surrounded by fairly steep cliffs but with one good landing place. The island had a number of well-built houses on it but had been abandoned by the inhabitants for economic reasons twelve years earlier. It belonged to the Duke of Sutherland who kindly lent it to us. A few of the houses were readily made habitable and early in July 1950 a party of twelve volunteers was, not unwillingly, marooned on the island. Most of them were students from the University of Aberdeen; in charge was an ex-superintendent of police. They were to be there for three months, their summer vacation, the longest period for which we could readily obtain volunteers. They took with them all the stores and equipment they needed for their stay; and they also had a small radio transmitter and receiver with which they maintained daily contact with the mainland.

One man had a cold on arrival, July 8th; another case occurred on July 9th and three more on July 11th. There were no more until the isolation ended on September 19th. On that day, a colleague and I landed and made contact with some of the party to see whether any stranger, even without a cold, could introduce infection. Nothing having happened, another of our team arrived with five others; all had just been inoculated in Aberdeen with one of our 'pedigree' colds, that is one which had been studied for some while at Salisbury. Meanwhile the island had been divided into three, each third inhabited by a party of four islanders, who kept apart from the other two parties. Each group was exposed under different conditions to the newly arrived party, each of whom had either developed a cold already, or did so very shortly after landing. The 'colds' had arrived late in the day, but as early colds are probably the most infectious we carried out the experiment forthwith and far into the night. It was a fine night and a magnificent display of the Aurora Borealis made the whole thing most romantic.

The six invaders with colds attempted to infect the islanders in one of three ways. They occupied a room in one of the houses for three hours in the absence of the four 'natives' (party A). To quote the report: 'During their occupation they were liberal in the way they disseminated nasal discharge on playing cards, books, cutlery and handles of cups, letters, chairs, door-handles and tables'. They then left the room, which was aired for half an hour before party A entered. The invaders then occupied a room with party B, being separated from them by a blanket stretched across the room but not quite reaching floor or ceiling. This arrangement was intended, and in fact shown by appropriate tests, to permit fine droplet nuclei to pass to the opposite half of the room while stopping coarse particles. Party C lived and ate with the people with the colds for three days, allowing maximum exposure. To our intense surprise and disappointment, no colds developed in any of the groups. Four more people with colds arrived a few days later and were exposed to party A under conditions of 'maximum exposure'. Again no colds developed.

We then learnt, through our radio, of a crofter on the mainland who had a cold, though not a very early, streaming one. He was exposed to party B, talking round a fire for two periods of two hours, and this time transfer was successful, three or four of the B's developed colds within a few days. In reviewing the results we inclined to think at the time that our 'pedigree' cold strain was for some reason less infective than a naturally occurring one. In the light of later work on the multiplicity of strains of cold-viruses it seems far more likely that the islanders were resistant as a result of the little outbreak of colds a few days after their isolation began; and that by bad luck this was due to a virus of the same type as the pedigree virus used in the later test.

Our comment on this curious episode is a little different from Sir Christopher's. Colds were not caught under the controlled circumstances, and we are therefore not forced to accept person-to-person transmission. Colds were caught only when a factor outside of what was known came to be introduced. Since the crofter on the nearby mainland contracted a cold, then according to our point of view, virus must have been falling close to the island itself within a few days of the meetings around the fire, possibly as an outcome of the magnificent display of the aurora.

In 1933, J. H. Paul and H. L. Freese published data from the island of Spitzbergen, and these are often quoted as giving proof of person-to-person transmission of the common cold. Colds largely died out during the Spitzbergen winter, when those remaining on the island were cut-off from the outside world. Then with the coming of the first boats in the spring an explosive increase in the number of colds occurred, and it was claimed that the islanders caught the disease from incoming migrants. This work is discrepant, however, not only with the experiment on Eilean nan Ron, but also from experience in the southern hemisphere. From Figure 3.2 it will be seen that for the three years 1965–1967 there was no epidemic at Tristan da Cunha following the arrival of the first boats in the southern-hemisphere spring. The lack of correlation with the winter temperature at Spitzbergen is also sharply different from the correlation found in Gloucestershire by Dr Hope-Simpson. The argument we gave previously to explain Dr Hope-Simpson's results fails, it is significant to note, for polar regions where the ocean becomes frozen or covered by pack-ice in winter. We think the melting of the sea in spring may well be the important physical phenomenon, leading to atmospheric disturbances which cause small micrometeorites to be pulled down from the stratosphere into the lower atmosphere. The first ships arrive in Spitzbergen at just the time when there is open water around the island. Indeed the arrival of the first ships is no more than a signal of the moment of melting of the sea. This is true not only for Spitzbergen but for other stations in the arctic and antarctic.

The survey of Paul and Freese was carried out among a population of Norwegians living almost wholly in Longyear City. There were fifty-one women and forty children in a total of 507, the great majority of the men being coal miners. The survey, which extended from 25 September 1930 to 10 August 1931, included the bacterial analysis of throat swabbings taken at three-monthly intervals from a sample of about one hundred and forty persons. Much of the original paper of Paul and Freese is concerned with this analysis, which in retrospect seems unfortunate because it revealed little difference among the sample, and little difference from the swabbings taken from those who arrived with the first boat in the spring of 1931. We would have preferred a discussion of how standards of diagnosis were maintained uniformly for an affliction as notoriously variable as the common cold, and especially of how this was done through the darkness of a Spitzbergen winter. On this evidently important issue, Paul and Freese offer no more than this:

> All medical service on the islands is in the hands of a capable young physician employed by the mining company, Dr John Friis. We had his wholehearted co-operation throughout our study. By means of regular personal visits to the townsfolk through daily conference with Dr Friis we obtained a fairly complete knowledge of all cases of respiratory diseases.

The boat which arrived at Longyear City on 31 May 1931 brought about fifty persons, who were examined before landing for respiratory illnesses. Two of the ship's crew were recovering from colds which had begun about a week previously, but Paul and Freese go on to tell us that these two had 'no direct contact with the town proper'. Within hours of landing, however, one of the new arrivals showed 'all the classical symptoms of a fresh cold'. We find it curious that no account is given in detail of the movements and contacts of this particular individual, who according to orthodox epidemiology was the most likely candidate for having caused the enormous outbreak of colds which followed among the inhabitants of Longyear City. Colds among the inhabitants began with three men, and of them Paul and Freese merely say: 'We were unable to trace any direct contact between the man with the cold who had arrived on the first boat and these three men.'

In no case where colds or influenza is supposed to have been 'brought' to an isolated community from the outside world have we found details given of the contacts responsible for the 'bringing' of the disease. As with Paul and Freese, there is always a prime candidate, but the candidate is a shadow without face and without name. This individual, a 'supershedder' of virus, is in our view an invention, modelled rather obviously on the medieval figure of death.

We add a more mundane comment. Household dust, if it contains an organism known as the house mite, readily causes fits of allergy. The overcrowded conditions mentioned by Paul and Freese for the Spitzbergen experiment of 1931 could have been conducive to the breeding of the house mite. If the melting of pack-ice, followed by the arrival of the first boat of the year, was also a signal for intensive spring cleaning throughout Longyear City, then likely enough there would have been allergic sneezing all over the town. Allergy was much less understood in 1931 than it is today, and it does not seem to us implausible that allergic attacks were added into Figure 3.3.

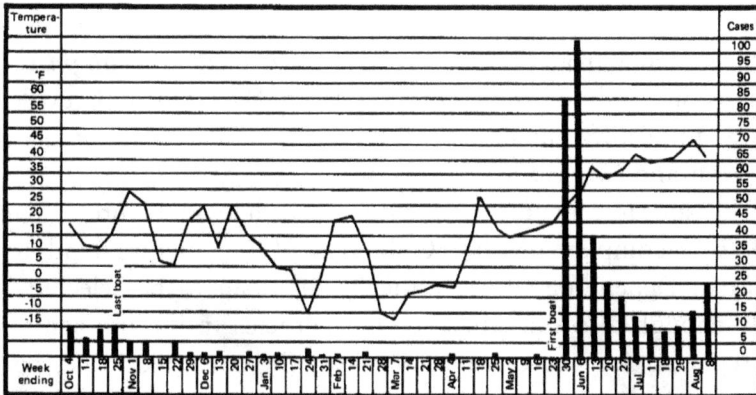

Fig. 3.3. Incidence of the common cold in Spitzbergen. The curve indicates temperature and the vertical black columns the number of colds occurring each week (from J. H. Paul and H. L. Freese, *American Journal of Hygiene*, 17, 517, 1933).

Modern investigations in the antarctic, when interpreted with respect to the orthodox theory of transmission of the common cold, are quite variable in their implications. M. J. Hohnes, T. R. Allen, A. F. Bradburne and E. J. Stott detail the movements of the RRS *John Briscoe*, with respect to outbreaks of upper respiratory illness on both the boat itself and following its arrival at the British base at Stonington Island. These data agree well with orthodox theory. On the other hand, A. S. Cameron and B. W. Moore, reporting on the wintering-over of men at the Australian base of Mawson, arrive at the remarkable conclusion that these men had a *less* than normal tendency to catch colds: 'These observations suggest that there is a reduced susceptibility to colds in many wintering-over parties while still on ice, though exceptions have been recorded.'

The exception which Cameron and Moore choose to quote is contrary to the usual epidemiologic claims, such as those of Paul and Freese, as well as to the data of Holmes, Allen, Bradburne and Stott: '... an experience recounted by Dr Goldsmith concerning members of a wintering party from Halley Bay, many of whom caught severe colds on boarding the relief ship.' So far so good for orthodox theory. But now: 'Several days later, however, these men, still suffering from their colds, came in contact with another wintering party from Shackleton Base, *none of whom caught colds.*' This second half of the quotation from Dr Goldsmith evidently puts a quite different complexion on the situation referred to by Cameron and Moore.

The sporadic incidence of virus according to Figure 2.3 must lead to a complex picture. Only bits of the picture tend to be reported. Depending on how the bits happen to be selected, and likely enough also on subjective inaccuracies in the moments that are reported for the onset of illnesses (in our experience, people differ by at least two days in the moments at which they 'give in' to a cold), it is possible to make almost any argument one pleases. Accuracy depends on the whole picture being available, and on every victim being under continuous clinical observation requirements that are almost impossible to satisfy under difficult field conditions.

To sum up the position, the evidence against person-to-person transmission of the common cold is suggestive but not decisive, and indeed many will continue to regard Figure 3.3 as demonstrating that transmission does take place, at least in special circumstances. Yet in every instance where person-to-person transmission might have been proved unequivocally, the attempted proof has demonstrated the opposite situation, namely that transmission did not take place (as for instance on Eilean nan Ron). We ourselves believe that theories which fail to prove themselves, in spite of being given repeated opportunities to do so, are to be viewed with suspicion.

4
History of a Disease

The somewhat scattered and diverse facts concerning influenza that will be reviewed in this chapter first convinced us that the idea of diseases from space must be taken seriously. We shall also deal with influenza in the two following chapters, where we come to a more definitive discussion which we regard as proving the correctness of the main ideas of this book.

Influenza, like the common cold, is a respiratory disease that appears to be continuously driven from outside the Earth. The pathogenic reservoir for influenza seems to be replenished on the time-scale of a few years. Unlike the common cold, however, influenza is a serious illness with the alarming possibility of severe complication, and often with unacceptably high risks of fatality. For instance, deaths due to influenza during 1918 are thought to have at least equalled the fatalities in the Great War itself. For this reason, public health authorities take influenza pandemics very seriously, and consequently there is considerably more recorded information for influenza than there is for the common cold.

The clinical symptoms of influenza and its mode of incidence on human communities are sufficiently distinctive for the disease to be identified from historical descriptions. The onset of influenza is sudden, the first symptoms being a headache and a general, non-specific feeling of illness. Within a few hours the body temperature rises often to above 101°F and there is a dry non-productive cough. Aching of muscles, mainly of the back and limbs, is a common feature and there is often accompanying pain in the joints. The disease normally runs a favourable course. The fever usually lasts for only three days, but an aftermath of lassitude and tiredness can persist over a much longer period of convalescence. Possible complications include the sudden onset of pneumonia, which is more likely to happen when an influenza outbreak is on a worldwide pandemic level.

It is an important and characteristic feature of influenza that outbreaks occur simultaneously across extensive tracts of country. This phenomenon of simultaneous attack led distinguished medical men to maintain for a long time that influenza cannot be transmitted by person-to-person infection. Indeed, the name influenza was introduced in Italy in the fifteenth century to describe an epidemic that was thought to arise from the influence of the stars. The earliest medical record of influenza-like disease is given by Hippocrates in 412 BC, though the identification with influenza is questionable in this instance. The first medically recorded epidemic of influenza occurred in Italy, Germany and England in 1173.

The condition known as the 'English Sweats', which came in five epidemics between 1485 and 1552, was probably a lethal variety of influenza. Millions of people are thought to have died of this disease. Symptoms included sweats, fever, vomiting and thirst. As in the case of influenza, one attack did not always confer immunity against subsequent attacks. Thousands of people are said to have suffered several successive bouts of illness. The condition is believed to have been first detected in London, but it was undoubtedly present in other European countries during this time. Then in 1552 the disease disappeared as mysteriously as it had appeared.

The symptoms of influenza are clearly seen in a letter which Lord Randolph sent from Edinburgh addressed to Lord Cecil in November 1562:

> Maybe it please your Honor, immediately upon the Quene's [Mary] arrival here, she fell acquaynted with a new disease that is common in this towne, called here the newe acquayntance, which passed also through her whole courte neither sparinge lordes, ladies nor damoysells not so much as ether Frenche or English. It ys a plague in their heades that have yet, and a sorenes in their stomackes, with a great coughe, that remayneth with some longer, with others

shorter time, as yet findeth apte bodies for the nature of the disease. The queen kept her bed six days. There was no appearance of danger, nor manie that die of the disease, excepte some old folkes. My lord of Murraye is now presently in it, the lord of Lidlington hathe had it, and I am ashamed to say that I have byne free of it, seinge it seketh acquayntance at all man's handes.

The first well-documented influenza pandemic occurred in 1580. This pandemic had a presumed origin in Asia and spread from there quickly to Africa, Europe and America. Mortality was high in many cities and amounted to thousands of deaths daily. It is said to have been of such intense virulence that 'in the space of six weeks it afflicted almost all the nations of Europe, of whom hardly the twentieth person was free of the disease... Its sudden ending after a month, as if it had been prohibited, was as marvellous as its sudden onset.'

Details of influenza pandemics for the years 1600 to 1900 are not very accurate, but Professor W. I. B. Beveridge has recently analysed many sources of historical data and finds seven certain pandemics and nine possible pandemics on record for the years 1700 to 1900 (see Table 4.1). The term 'influenza' seems to have come into common English usage during the European pandemic of 1743.

For the forty years before 1889 the sporadic appearance of influenza pandemics was evidently not uncommon, according to Professor Beveridge's table. There is general agreement, however, that during this period, influenza was a relatively harmless disease and caused few deaths, at any rate in Britain. (It is interesting to note that the death-rate from influenza, even during its 'harmless' period, was still considerably larger than the death-rate that has been estimated to result from an all-nuclear energy economy.) Figure 4.1 shows the annual death-rate from influenza per 100,000 in England and Wales during the period 1860–1948. It is noteworthy that 1890 marks a sudden step function rise in the death-rate, a rise from which we have never since quite recovered. A satisfactory reason for this steep rise has not been given, but a

Table 4.1. *Influenza pandemics 1700–1900* (after W. I. B. Beveridge).

Certain	Possible
—	1729–30
1732–33	—
—	1742–43
—	1761–62
—	1767
—	1775–76
1781–82	—
—	1788–89
1800–02	—
1830–33	—
—	1836–37
1847–48	—
—	1850–51
1857–58	—
—	1873–75
1889–90	—

possible explanation could be that the years 1889–1890 marked the advent from space of new influenza types possessing suddenly increased degrees of virulence.

The first outbreaks of the 1889 pandemic occurred in Bukhara in Russia in May and June of that year. By October, influenza had spread to Tomsk in Siberia and to Leningrad (St Petersburg), and by November and December the whole of Western Europe and North America were engulfed. During the following four to six months the entire world population was involved with high attack-rates and high mortality everywhere.

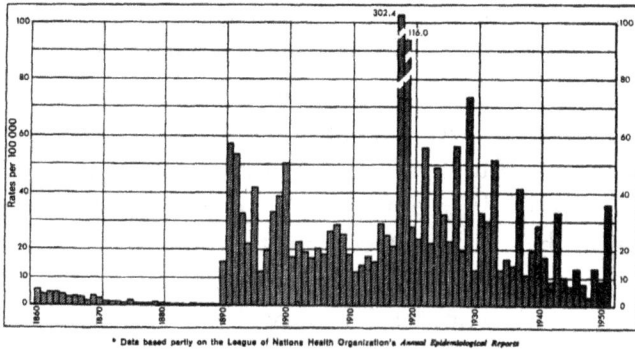

* Data based partly on the League of Nations Health Organization's *Annual Epidemiological Reports*

Fig. 4.1. Annual death-rate from influenza in England and Wales (from *Influenza: A Review of Current Research,* WHO Monograph Series, 1954).

Perhaps the most disastrous influenza pandemic on record occurred in 1917–1919. Estimates of the death toll vary from a minimum of twenty million people to about twice that number. There are some estimates which suggest that twenty million deaths occurred in India alone, and in parts of Alaska and the Pacific Islands over half the total population in certain villages and cities died. The situation as it occurred in Alaska, under conditions when ground transportation had become essentially impossible, is described in Chapter 7. There were three waves of pandemic influenza in less than twelve months. In the first wave, which occurred in the spring of 1918, the proportion of people attacked averaged about fifty per cent but the mortality was fortunately not high. The second wave, which came in the autumn, was also characterised by high attack-rates and in this second wave there was high mortality, deaths being mainly in the 20–40 age group. The third wave, which followed early in 1919, was somewhat less severe, but again a disconcerting preponderance of healthy young persons was affected.

The scale of the disaster caused by the 1917–1919 pandemic is hard to visualise. Many cities and villages were almost completely depopulated in a matter of weeks. In the State of Punjab, streets were strewn with the dead bodies of victims, and at railway stations trains had to be continually cleared of dead or dying passengers. As with other influenza pandemics, both earlier and later, there were some gross and inexplicable inconsistencies in the behaviour of the influenza virus. St Helena, an island in mid-Atlantic, is known to have definitely escaped, despite all the shipping that must have called there. Then there was a puzzling long delay before the pandemic reached Australia. This country seems to have been quite remarkably free of disease until early in 1919, despite all the ships which pull in there from infected ports, and despite all the attacks which occurred in mid-ocean. The first influenza death in Australia occurred at Sydney on 10 February 1919 and was reported in *The Times* of London of 20 February 1919. It was claimed that this amazing postponement was due to the imposition of strict quarantine by Australian port authorities. Quarantine, however, has not otherwise been found effective for influenza, nor could it have been enforced to a degree that was complete enough to result in the abeyance of the disease. (Medical reports from Australia, appearing in *The Lancet* in late 1919, suggest that the quarantine claims had been much exaggerated by a bureaucracy anxious to defend itself against widespread criticism.)

Again there were glaring inequalities in the way ships at sea were affected. Passenger liners arriving in Australia during the pandemic recorded attack-rates aboard ship that varied between four and forty-three per cent. And there were similar differences in the attack-rates on crews of ships in the British Navy. There were also gross differences in the behaviour of English public schools, an issue which we shall take up in detail in Chapter 6.

The highly erratic behaviour of the influenza virus, which was thus brought home so dramatically in the 1917–1919 pandemic, is hard to reconcile with the usual orthodox idea of a person-to-person spread of the disease. The virus apparently has the property of being able to make leaps in days over many thousand miles on the one hand, and is yet barely able to travel tens of miles in periods of weeks or months. This is how Dr Louis Weinstein writes of the 1917–1919 pandemic:

The influenza pandemic of 1918 occurred in three waves. The first appeared in the winter and spring of 1917–18... This wave was characterised by high attack rates (50 per cent of the world's population was affected) but by very low fatality rates... The lethal second wave, which started at Ford Devens in Ayer, Massachusetts, on September 12, 1918, involved almost the entire world over a very short time... Its epidemiologic behaviour was most unusual. Although person-to-person spread occurred in local areas, the disease appeared on the same day in widely separated parts of the world on the one hand, but, on the other, took days to weeks to spread relatively short distances. It was detected in Boston and Bombay on the same day, but took three weeks before it reached New York City, despite the fact that there was considerable travel between the two cities. It was present for the first time at Joliet in the State of Illinois *four weeks* after it was first detected in Chicago, the distance between those areas being only 38 miles...

The lethal second wave of the 1918 pandemic also provided evidence of local patchiness from one American city to another. Death-rates from respiratory disease in the late months of 1918 were remarkably variable between different cities. A striking contrast came from Pittsburg and Toledo, neighbouring cities with normally almost identical death-rates, and with populations of similar age groupings that are concerned with similar daily occupations. The late-1918 death-rate from respiratory diseases in Pittsburg exceeded that in Toledo, not by a few per cent or a few tens of per cent, but by an enormous 400 per cent.

Moving on thirty years to 1948, the influenza pandemic of that year began in Sardinia, spreading out from the initial region of incidence in the way shown in Figure 4.2. Because it was the initial focus, the situation as it occurred in Sardinia was the subject of careful subsequent study. Commenting on the first appearance of the disease, Professor F. Magrassi had this to say:

We were able to verify ... the appearance of influenza in shepherds who were living for a long time alone, in solitary open country far from any inhabited centre; this occurred absolutely contemporaneously with the appearance of influenza in the nearest inhabited centres.

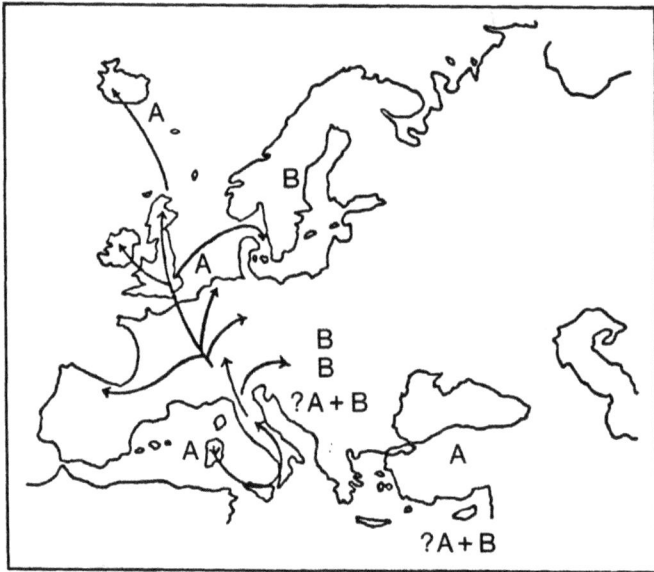

Fig. 4.2. Spread of 1948 influenza epidemic from a presumed focus in Sardinia (from C. Andrewes, *The Common Cold,* Weidenfeld and Nicholson, London, 1965).

This type of evidence, and that which had inevitably become emphasised during the 1917–1919 pandemic, was not particularly new. For several centuries those doctors who were careful observers of natural phenomena had noticed the rapid spread of influenza during epidemics, a speed of spread that was inconsistent with any possible form of person-to-person transmission. As recently as 1894 the distinguished British epidemiologist, Charles Creighton, maintained that influenza was not an infectious disease. Citing medical opinion during the epidemic of 1833, 1837 and 1847, which held that the disease affected the entire country during the same one or two weeks, Creighton suggested that influenza was due to a 'miasma' spreading over the land rather than a disease that must spread by passing from person-to-person. The rejection of Creighton's position — despite all the evidence in his favour — seems to border on irrationality. Creighton was not taken seriously in the present century because, as M. W. Kaplan and R. G. Webster remark: 'By the end of the 19th Century ... the microbiological concept of infectious disease had taken firm root ...'

Strictly speaking, the microbiological concept requires only that victims of the disease should acquire the influenza virus from outside of themselves, which of course they would do if the invasion came from space. Such an idea, however, seemed so much less plausible to medical opinion than the concept of person-to-person transmission that it was not even considered as a hypothesis to be tested. It became an axiom.

The search for the causative agent of influenza was a long and difficult one. Throughout the period of the 1917–1919 pandemic there were many heroic volunteers who subjected themselves to filtered inoculants extracted from tissues of victims in fatal cases. Some transmissions were recorded but these were not considered significant in establishing the 'filter passer' or virus hypothesis. For some years after 1920 a bacillus known as Pfeiffer's influenza bacillus remained a leading candidate for the causative agent of influenza, but this identification was eventually proved wrong.

A close connection between human and animal influenza was already established in the fall of 1918. J. S. Koen, a veterinarian working at Fort Dodge, Iowa, reported that a new disease had appeared in pigs in the Middle West that was strikingly similar to human influenza. There was a similar report, which will be quoted at the end of this chapter, from a veterinary surgeon at Kirkby Stephen in Westmorland, but for sheep not pigs. Moreover, the disease in pigs had occurred contemporaneously with the attacks of influenza among farm families in the area. After many a frustrated attempt to demonstrate the transmissibility of influenza in pigs, using filtered mucous fluid from infected pigs, R. E. Shope showed in 1928 that such transmission was possible. A viral agent for pig influenza was thus clearly demonstrated. Filtered throat washings from infected human patients were shown in 1933 by Wilson Smith, C. H. Andrewes and P. P. Laidlaw to be capable of inducing influenza in ferrets.

In 1940, F. M. Burnet found that the influenza virus could be cultivated by injecting it into a developing chick embryo. Fertilised hen eggs that have incubated for ten days are inoculated with virus. After two or three further days of incubation, one could obtain ten thousand million virus particles in a few millilitres of fluid. Shortly afterwards it was shown that the virus so cultivated caused red blood cells to agglutinate or clump together, and that the serum of the blood could contain antibodies against a particular influenza virus that would prevent such clumping. (Possession of an appropriate antibody forms the basis of immunity against a particular virus.) Studies of clumping red blood cells in the presence of various antibodies were seen to provide means for classifying the various forms of the influenza virus, an idea that has now led to extensive microscopic as well as serological investigations of the virus.

One of the first facts to be discovered was that there are three different types of the virus, types A, B and C. All three have a similar appearance under the electron microscope, but their behaviour with respect to antibodies is quite different. Type C is relatively uncommon and unimportant and may be excluded from our discussion. Type A causes widespread epidemics and pandemics and is (at least at present) the most important. This is also the only influenza type that we share with pigs, horses and birds. Type B causes localised epidemics mainly amongst school children. Within type A itself there are a large number of variants known as subtypes.

Under an electron microscope, a type A influenza virus particle appears as a sphere approximately 100 nanometres in diameter, with radial 'spikes' emerging from a number of places on the surface. These spikes are of two kinds. One combines with red blood cells, and causes them to clot or agglutinate, whereas the other acts in the opposite way, by breaking the bond between the virus particle and the red blood cell. The former type of spike, or antigen, is called haemaglutinin (H), and the latter is called neuraminidase (N). It is H that is responsible for the attack, while N enables the virus to gain egress from an invaded cell, thereby permitting the virus to continue the attack. Following an influenza infection, antibodies are produced in the blood serum against both these H and N antigens, and the antibodies differentiate the several strains of influenza virus, as we have just discussed above. Encased within the spiked outer sphere of the virus are eight separated strands of genetic material, which act rather like separate chromosomes, generating separate proteins when the virus is in the process of attacking a host cell.

Influenza viruses are classified with respect to the H and N antigens. Whenever a new antigen appears, it is given the next number appearing on one or other of the series:

$$H0, H1, H2, H3 \ldots \text{ for the H-antigen,}$$
$$N1, N2, N3 \qquad \ldots \text{ for the N-antigen.}$$

The first human influenza virus to be isolated in 1933 was designated $H0\,N1$. A variant isolated in 1946 was designated $H1\,N1$, because there was a significant change in H but not in N.

The influenza virus is found to change slowly over the years — a process known as antigenic drift. Occasionally, however, dramatic changes occur (antigenic shifts) and such changes give rise to major new pandemics. The first major variant isolated after 1933 was $H2\,N2$ in the Asian flu epidemic of 1957, where both H and N antigens were found to have undergone shifts. Whereas antigenic drift can be attributed to the host developing immunity to a prevalent strain, major antigenic shifts are more difficult to understand within orthodox views. A theory which is currently in vogue appears to have been suggested by the discovery of influenza A in pigs, horses and birds. A hybrid genetic cross, of a kind that was shown possible in the laboratory by F. M. Burnet and P. E. Lind, is postulated to occur under natural conditions, the cross taking place between a human virus and an animal virus. A subclinical spread of the new virus is then postulated, with the further requirement that the virus is later shocked into 'virulence' in the human population by some natural event. We shall return to their theory in the next chapter.

The distribution of the H and N antigens of the influenza A virus known to be, or to have been, present in man and other animals is shown in Table 4.2. The large number of antigenic variants amongst birds is worthy of note. It would seem entirely natural that other animals should tend to be attacked by the same invading pathogens as ourselves. For respiratory diseases, birds are especially vulnerable to attack, because they sample the air more widely than do land-based animals. If the attack on the Earth is patchy, birds would inevitably tend to find the pathogenic patches, whereas land animals may often escape them.

During major pandemics we would expect animals to be affected contemporaneously with attacks on humans.

We have already noted that during the 1917–1919 pandemic this was so for pigs in the United States. There is also evidence to indicate that large numbers of monkeys and baboons in South Africa died contemporaneously with the human pandemic. Since baboons are not domestic animals, and human–baboon contact must be virtually non-existent, this was clearly a case of an independent attack on creatures other than ourselves. During the 1917–1919 pandemic, large numbers of moose, bison, elk and buffaloes are reported to have died in Canada and the United States, and large numbers of sheep died in England. We end this chapter with the following quotation from *The Lancet* of 19 March 1919:

Does epidemic influenza affect the lower animals?

In former days there was a general impression that influenza when epidemic in man spread to some of the lower animals, such as the horse, for example. In more recent times this view was considered to be untenable, and it has to be admitted that little evidence of any scientific value has ever been brought forward to support the contention that any of the domestic animals were susceptible to the disease. During the course of the present pandemic the question has again been raised, chiefly in the lay press. A Central News message, published in a London newspaper on Nov. 1st, 1918, from Johannesburg, mentioned that 'an extraordinary development' of the influenza epidemic, then raging in South Africa, had been the excessive mortality that had occurred among the African monkeys. Reports from areas in which these animals abounded

Table 4.2.   Subtypes of influenza A[*].

Host	Place and Year First Isolated	H	N
Man	England, 1933	0	1
Man	Australia, 1946	1	1
Man	Singapore, 1957	2	2
Man	Hong Kong, 1968	3	2
Man	New Jersey, 1976	1	1
Swine	Iowa, 1930	1	1
Swine	Taiwan, 1970	3	2
Horse	Prague, 1956	eq 1 (av 1)	eq 1
Horse	Miami, 1963	eq 2 (3)	eq 2
Chicken	Indonesia, 1927	av 1 (eq 1)	eq 1
Chicken	Rostock, 1934	av 1 (eq 1)	1
Chicken	Germany, 1949	av 2	eq 1
Duck	England, 1956	av 3	av 1
duck	Czechoslovakia, 1956	av 4	av 1
Chicken	Scotland, 1959	av 5 (1)	1
Tern	South Africa, 1961	av 5 (1)	av 2
Turkey	Canada, 1963	av 6 (3)	eq 2
Duck	Ukraine, 1963	av 7 (3, eq 2)	eq 2
Turkey	England, 1963	av 1 (eq 1)	av 3
Turkey	Mass, USA, 1965	av 6	2
Quail	Italy, 1965	av 2	eq 2
Duck	Italy, 1966	av 2	2
Duck	Germany, 1968	av 6	1
Turkey	Ontario, 1968	av 8	av 4
Shearwater	Queensland, 1971	av 6	av 5
Duck	Germany, 1973	2	av 2
Duck	Tennessee, USA, 1974	av 3	av 6

eq = equine,   av = avian
[*]From W. I. B. Beveridge, *Influenza, the last great plague*, W. H. Heinemann, London, 1977.

stated that the monkeys were 'dying in hundreds', and that in some places whole troops of baboons had been found dead, the result apparently of 'pneumonic complications.' These statements were supplemented by the Cape Town correspondent of *The Times* on Nov. 5th, who said that influenza had spread to baboons, of which a large number existed in the kloofs and hills around Magaliesburg, in the Transvaal. These animals were 'dying in scores' and their dead bodies were being found on the roadsides and in the vicinity of homesteads, the epidemic having apparently led them to forsake their usual haunts. Recent experiments in France, conducted by British research workers, have proved that influenza can be transmitted to monkeys by the inoculation of infective material; so that it may be concluded that these animals are susceptible to the disease, but whether they can contract it also in the natural way is not yet clear. Reports from Canada, at the end of 1918, stated that woodmen employed in clearing the bush in Northern Ontario had observed an unusual mortality among moose; and this they believed to be due to the current influenza epidemic. *The Times* of Jan. 10th supports this statement and says that in Northern Canada influenza was 'decimating the big game', and that for some time smaller animals had also shown marked symptoms of the disease. *The Times* of Feb. 20th contains a communication from its correspondent at Butte, Montana, mentioning the fact that the Yellowstone National Park, in which bison, elk, and other animals are strictly preserved by the United States Government, had been 'swept by an epidemic of influenza', and that already 31 'buffaloes' had been found dead as a result. On March 10th it was reported by *The Times* that a veterinary surgeon [Mr Malloch] at Kirkby Stephen, who was inspecting officer for the Westmorland County Council and for the Board of Agriculture, had lately observed an epidemic illness among sheep in the district, and that he had diagnosed it as 'influenza'; it was also stated that this veterinary surgeon during his 30 years of professional life had never, till now, met with an outbreak of a similar kind. Several flocks were at present affected, and many sheep had died as a result of the epidemic.

5
Spread of a Virus

According to our theory, which is that bacteria and viruses are incident from space, some diseases will be infectious and others will not. On the usual view, however, which requires every disease to have a permanent pathogenic reservoir indigenous to the Earth, diseases are always 'caught', either through person-to-person transmission or through a transfer from animal to human. For influenza, there is no known permanent human reservoir, and so it is usual to postulate that one or more of the reservoirs existing in the animals of Table 4.2 can emerge from time to time in an assault on the human population. Emergence is thought to be associated with two different subtypes of virus coming together in an animal host cell, and with their genetic material becoming mixed during replication in a viable way, thereby producing a new active subtype of virus distinct from its two parents. It may happen that humans are susceptible to the new subtype. If so, it is argued, the new subtype bursts out of its animal host into the human population, like a snake breaking out from a hitherto closed box.

The generation of new subtypes of virus through hybrid cross is known to be possible, as we mentioned already in Chapter 4. Although the process may be common in animals, cases in which the new recombinant hybrid happens to be highly pathogenic for man must be uncommon. Hence we cannot postulate that a new subtype, virulent for man, emerges simultaneously in many different geographical places. There must be just one focus of emergence of the new subtype, which must then spread out from the single focus by transmission. The emergence from a focus, as it is supposed to have occurred in 1957, is shown in Figure 5.1. This was the so-called 'Asian flu' of subtype H2 N2.

Unlike this 'snake out of box' theory, for a pathogenic invader from space the H2 N2 subtype would be incident all over the Earth. There would, however, be a dispersion in time of its arrival at ground level, because of latitude variations in the height of the troposphere, because of the capricious nature of eddy transfers between the troposphere and the stratosphere (and also within the stratosphere itself), and because of local variations in storm activity causing complex electric field patterns in the upper atmosphere. The months of the year marked in circles on Figure 5.1 simply give the times of arrival at ground level of the infalling pathogen. From this point of view, the arrows of Figure 5.1 have no relevance.

Are the arrows of Figure 5.1 really very sensible anyway? Did the virus really need four whole months to travel from Japan and Hong Kong along the busy air routes into Europe? The time dispersion of Figure 5.1 is generally comparable with that of the pandemics of former times, which of course it should be for a virus incident from space. Of the 1889–1890 pandemic, Professor Beveridge writes:

> This was the so-called Asiatic influenza pandemic. The first report was from Bukhara in Russia in May. At the start it spread very slowly and it was not until October that it reached Tomsk and the Caucasus. Then it spread rapidly westward and throughout the world.

Plainly the spread of influenza ignores the technology of human travel, as we can see more clearly from the detailed incidence of the 1968 pandemic (H3 N2) mapped on to the United States. Influenza outbreaks on a state-by-state basis over a period of twelve weeks are shown in Figure 5.2. This was the so-called Hong Kong flu. Because California is the nearest US State to Hong Kong, it might seem natural that the first US outbreak should have occurred in California. It is decidedly less natural, however, that the first California outbreak should have occurred in the small desert town

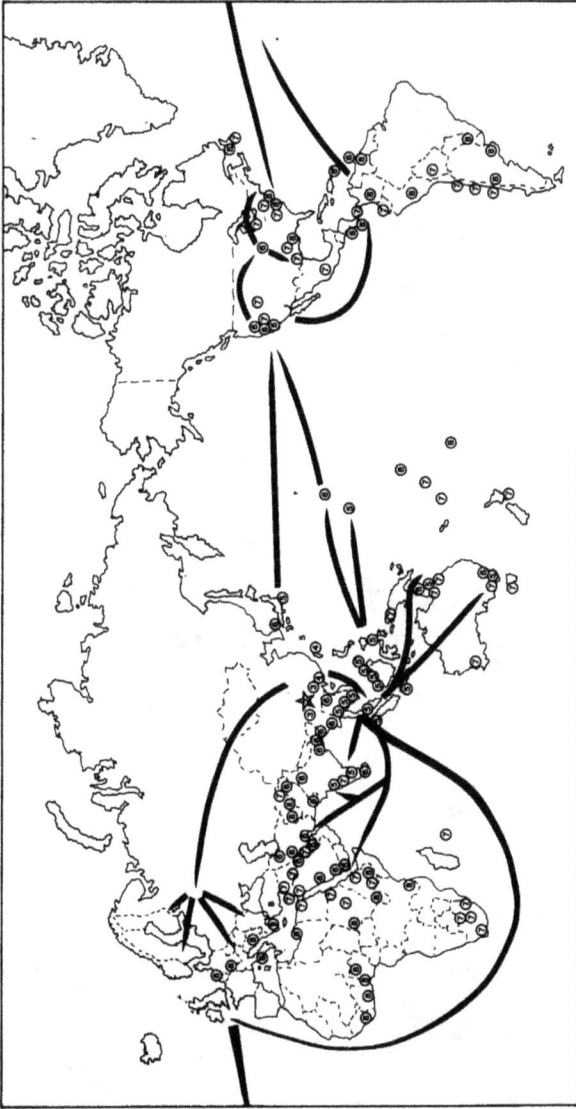

Fig. 5.1. The behaviour of the 1957 Asian flu pandemic,
② = Presumed origin of epidemic at second month of year,
⑥ = Epidemic at the sixth month of year,
(From C. H. Stuart-Harris and G. C. Schjld, *Influenza*, E. Arnold, 1976).

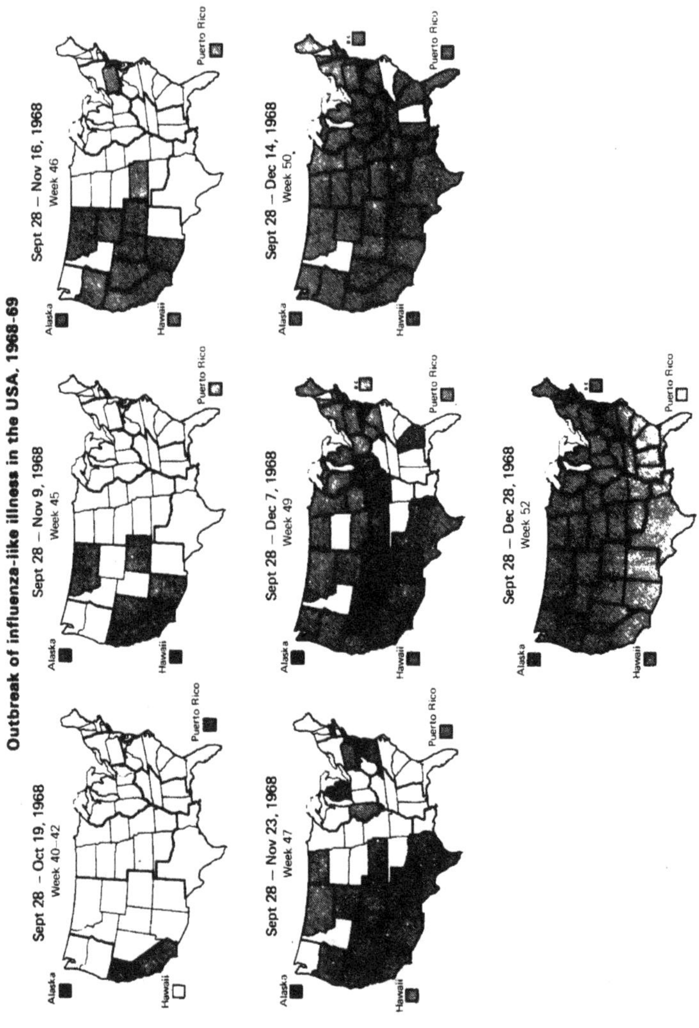

Fig. 5.2. State-by-state spread of influenza during the 1968 epidemic (from *Influenza-Virus, Vaccines, Strategy,* ed. P. Selby, Academic Press, 1976).

of Needles, not in a large population centre such as Los Angeles, San Diego or San Francisco. By week 45 the disease had spread into the adjoining states of Nevada, Arizona and Colorado. It had also made a leap, not along the popular air routes to New York or Chicago, but to Montana. Week 46 shows a further stepwise filling-in among the mountain states; and at last, six weeks from the first outbreak, there is a leap to New York, but still not to Chicago, or to Dallas or to Miami. By week 47 a patch in the north-east is filling out, Chicago has it, and Texas has joined the West. Week 49 is interesting for the circumstance that the well-known intensive November–December holiday traffic from the north-east to Florida has still not infected Miami. While boats have allegedly carried influenza with uncanny speed, aircraft clearly do not. The pattern of Figure 5.2 is plainly geographic. The disease hit first at the Pacific and mountain states. The next focus hit the north-east and the Great Lakes area. The last to be reached was the south-east. All this is consistent with an infall of the influenza virus from space, and with weather patterns and local meteorological conditions causing geographic variations in the time of infall.

There were surprises for the recombinant virus theory in both 1957 and 1968, a circumstance that has recently been repeated in a sharpened form (1977). In 1958, J. Mulder and N. Masurel published in *The Lancet* a communication entitled 'Pre-epidemic antibodies against the 1957 strain of Asian influenza virus in the serum of older persons living in the Netherlands'. What Mulder and Masurel found was that blood samples taken before 1957 from old people, who in 1957 were in the age range 75–85, had high concentrations of antibodies to the Asian virus (H2 N2). Younger people did not have the same high concentrations. The inference was that old people must have encountered the same virus subtype, but seventy-five years or so earlier. It was suggested that the 1889–1890 pandemic might have been H2 N2. but since 1957 minus 1889 is only 68 years, it seems better to suppose that the H2 N2 was incident in a smaller outbreak than that of 1889–1890, an outbreak occurring around 1880.

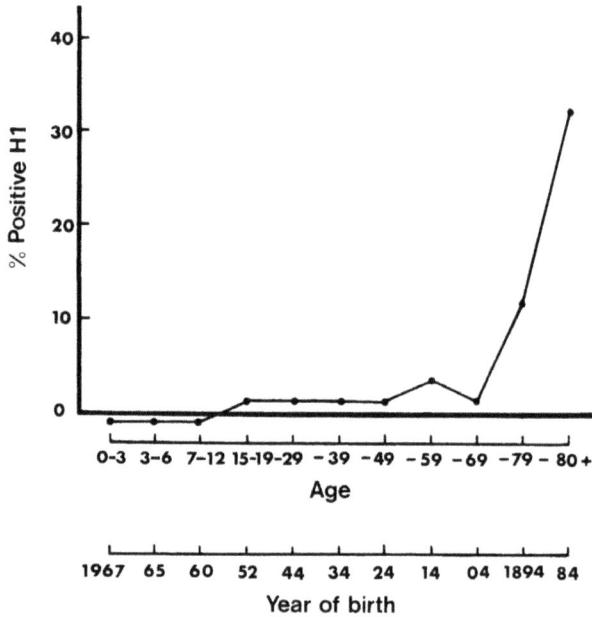

Fig. 5.3. Age distribution of 1/30 positive antibody titres to Asian Flu, *before* an epidemic in 1957 (plotted from data in S. J. Machin *et al.*, *Journal of Hygiene,* Cambridge, 68, 497).

The same interval of 75–80 years appeared again for the H3 N2 pandemic of 1968. Figure 5.3 shows the presence of antibodies to this subtype in blood samples collected before the pandemic occurred. These results, obtained by S. J. Machin, C. W. Potter and J. S. Oxford, show a moderate rise above the estimated zero level for the age group 69–79, followed by a far more marked rise in the age group 79–80+. The strong implication of Figure 5.3 is that the virus subtype responsible for the 1889–1890 pandemic was H3 N2; or if several subtypes were involved in this pandemic, H3 N2 was among them.

The phenomenon of the recombinant cross of two subtypes of virus, to produce a third subtype different from the parents, should not lead back to the original subtypes, except as a fluke of great rarity. Yet here were two subtypes (H2 N2 and H3 N2) apparently repeating themselves. On the other hand there is good reason to expect that after an interval of years, the Earth might encounter the same cloud of micrometeorites. The latter, being derived from comets, have eccentric orbits around the Sun with periodicities that are mostly quite different from (longer than) that of the Earth itself. Micrometeorites from the same comet tend to extend in a ribbon-like distribution along their orbit. Depending on the amount of this extension, encounters with the Earth can vary from twice a year to being exceedingly infrequent. For a compact cloud of meteorites, if encounter is to take place, the Earth must not only cross the orbit of the cloud but it must do so at just the moment when the cloud happens to be at the crossing point. This will happen only very rarely, because of the so-called incommensurability of the orbital periods of the Earth and the meteorites. As the cloud spreads itself more and more into a ribbon, however, it will take longer and longer for all the meteorites to pass through the region of the crossing point, giving an increasing chance for the Earth to arrive there while the meteorites are still passing by. Indeed, with sufficient spreading, it will take longer than a year for the whole distribution of meteorites to sweep through the region of the crossing point, and then encounter will be certain to occur, every time the elongated cluster of meteorites goes around its orbit. For micrometeorites containing bacteria and viruses we can therefore have repeated encounters with the same pathogen. The interval of 75 to 80 years for both H2 N2 and H3 N2 suggests a connection with Halley's comet, which has a present-day period of 76.2 years, but which has varied over the past two millennia from about 75 years on the low side to about 79 years on the high side.

This is our first mention of an explicit comet, and it may be wondered why we have not sought to develop our point of view in terms of a roster of comets, giving dates when the Earth has actually crossed their paths, and then correlating the outbreaks of disease with the known encounters. But comets do not shed just one cloud of micrometeorites. From a particular comet there will be several, perhaps many, such clouds and each one of them will behave in the manner discussed above. Moreover, the several clouds of micrometeorites come to follow different orbits, because they are disturbed in different ways by the gravitational fields of the planets. Nor would such clouds continue to follow the same orbit as the parent comet. The problem is therefore one of extreme complexity, to which there is no simple solution.

It is possible to examine with radar techniques meteors entering the Earth's atmosphere that are large enough to produce trails of ionised gas, and thence to determine what the orbits of the meteors were before they encountered the Earth. An analysis of 19,303 such trails obtained by the 6-station Radio Meteor Project at Havana, Illinois, has been reported by Z. Sekanina. Meteors from streams which are associated with comets were found, but with orbits that were considerably variable from the original comet, and variable from one another. This finding verifies directly the conclusion of the preceding paragraph. Cometary debris is therefore a complex mess.

Returning to the Asian flu virus of 1957 (H2 N2), and to the Hong Kong strain (H3 N2) of 1968, if indeed these subtypes reappeared after seventy-five to eighty years of abeyance, the usual theory of the recombinant origin of the antigenic shifts of the influenza virus is in trouble. The situation turns on the significance of the antibody content of the blood sera of old people (Figure 5.3). This might seem a somewhat thin basis on which to reject a widely held belief, and it is therefore of interest and importance that the same phenomenon has now arisen in a more direct way. The dominant strain of influenza virus from 1946 to 1957 was H1 N1 (see Table 4.2). After 1957, this particular subtype disappeared, only to reappear again in China in the Spring of 1977. Once again H1 N1 has now spread across much of the world. Here then we have a direct verification that influenza subtypes can disappear and reappear, which they should not do according to the recombinant hypothesis. There is no difficulty at all, however, from the point of view that influenza is a disease in man that is driven directly from space.

The best example known to us that is suggestive of a person-to-person transmission of influenza occurred on the island of Tristan da Cunha in August 1971. The epidemic involved 96 per cent of the 284 indigenous islanders. It followed immediately after the arrival of the boat *Tristania* on 13 August, as is shown in Figure 5.4. The boat had come from Cape Town, an eight-day journey. On it were five islanders who had visited Cape Town either for medical treatment or on holiday. Three of these five had come down with acute respiratory disease during the voyage and the other two did so shortly after landing. The boat crew itself was not affected. The alternative ways of explaining these facts are:

(1) A pathogenic patch of influenza virus hit Tristan da Cunha within a day or two of 13 August 1971. We have emphasised several times in preceding chapters that boats, because of their motion, are especially vulnerable to attack whenever their courses cross a region of incidence of patches of an infalling pathogen. Hence it would be likely for the *Tristania* to have been hit as well as the island itself.

(2) One or more of the visiting islanders picked up the virus, which was the Hong Kong subtype $H_3 N_2$, while in Cape Town. The virus was then 'kept going' through the eight-day voyage by being passed from one of the five islanders to another, and was still active at the time of the landing on 13 August. Once introduced into the island the epidemic exploded because the islanders had not hitherto been exposed to H3 N2, and therefore had no immunity (antibodies) against it.

The problem for the first of these alternatives is that, without there being a causal connection between the boat landing and the epidemic outbreak on the island, which occurred over the four days from 16 August to 19 August, we have to say that the boat landing on 13 August was coincidental in its timing. But this is not at all unlikely. From Figure 5.4, one can see that during the period in question boats landed on the island with an average frequency of about one to every eleven days, so that no very small chance would be involved in such a coincidence.

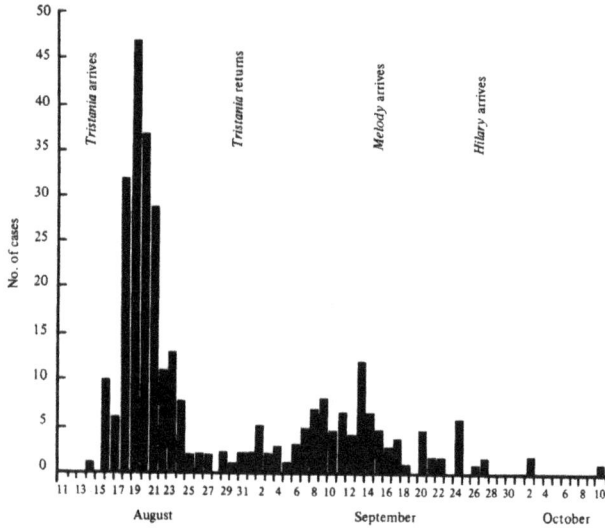

Fig. 5.4. Incidence of influenza in Tristan da Cunha (J. Mantle and D. A. J. Tyrrell, *Journal of Hygiene,* Cambridge, 71, 89, 1973).

The problems for the second explanation appear to us to be the more severe. First there is a discrepancy of the incubation periods. If the epidemic started with an islander picking up the virus in Cape Town before the *Tristania* sailed on 5 August, there must have been about ten days between this starting event and the time when the last of the five island travellers on the boat came down with clinical symptoms — and this occurred after the landing on 13 August. Yet the epidemic is supposed to have exploded on the island within only four days.

How did it come about, one can also ask, that Tristan da Cunha escaped the Hong Kong flu variant H3 N2, which appeared already in 1968, until 1971? Boats call frequently at the island, as we can sec in Figure 5.4, and as we saw in Chapter 3 in our discussion of outbreaks of common cold on this island. Tristan da Cunha is by no means isolated, and if the islanders had been like a tinder-box ready to flare up at the first spark, the spark would surely have been struck long before 1971. The escape of Tristan da Cunha for the three years from 1966 to 1971 is reminiscent of the escape of St Helena in the 1917–1919 pandemic, and clearly suggests that a meteorological influence generally helps in reducing the incidence of pathogenic attacks on mid-oceanic islands, at any rate islands in the South Atlantic.

When the first outbreaks of influenza began in Britain in December 1977 we began to wonder if some decisive test of the person-to-person transmission hypothesis could be made. We had in mind the carefully designed experiments of the Common Cold Research Unit at Salisbury, and we wondered if some such experiments could be made for influenza. Our first contacts with doctors of the Public Health Service made it clear that for ethical reasons clear-cut experiments were not possible. So we began to think of people who from the nature of their employment would be particularly exposed to attack. If there were person-to-person transmissions of the disease, then dentists and assistants and cashiers in department stores should be particularly vulnerable. Unfortunately, there was not enough time available in December 1977 to set up a properly designed enquiry, one that would stand up to the kind of criticism that we ourselves had made of data existing already in the medical literature. Table 5.1 illustrates what our worries were.

Table 5.1.

	Attack Rates %			
	Families		Individuals	
Groups	Lavender City	Grayville	Lavender City	Grayville
General Population	39	38	32	26
Physicians	56	52	34	33
Nurses	51	31	12	14
Pharmacists	15	33	7	17

Lavender City and Grayville were the two American towns selected by R. H. Drachman, G. M. Hochbaum and I. M. Rosenstock for a study of the incidence of the 1957 Asian flu (H2 N2). Both had populations of about 70,000, although only subsets of the total populations were actually involved in the survey (about 3000 in each city). By 'attack-rate' is meant the fraction, expressed as a per cent, that was diagnosed to have contracted the disease.

It is interesting that physicians when taken individually had attack-rates not much different from the general population, thereby showing that exposure to patients did not have any very obvious effect. On the other hand, the families of physicians displayed attack-rates far above the general population. Rejecting the hypothesis that the influenza virus has a special preference for the families of physicians, we decided that the effect was probably due to a non-uniform standard of diagnosis of the milder cases. Likewise we do not believe the virus distinguishes the special categories of nurses and pharmacists to anything like the degree that the numbers in Table 5.1 might suggest. We think that the table spells out the dangers of psychological factors entering into what must of necessity be a loose experiment. We believe that the low attack-rates on individual nurses are to be interpreted as showing that nurses are especially determined not to succumb to mild illnesses. Likewise pharmacists could well have been led into under-reporting their ailments through a determined belief in the efficacy of their wares.

Faced with Table 5.1, we decided against sending around questionnaires to department stores and to dentists. The fact that the public health authorities have never intervened to declare department stores and popular newsagents to be places of danger, and that — so far as we know — there has never been industrial action on behalf of workers in these places, suggested to us that among such workers there is no subjective feeling of being exposed to exceptional hazard.

There is an indication in the first line of Table 5.1 that members of families might be somewhat more susceptible to attack than persons living alone, implying a measure of person-to-person transmission, although the difference here could also be due to other factors — such as differences of age distribution, and of various correlations that we could think of in the reporting of marginal cases. It was clear, however, that effective tests of the transmission hypothesis could almost certainly be made by comparing families with individuals. If one were to take a set of young married couples in an influenza epidemic, some would turn out to be entirely unaffected, some would have a single spouse affected, and some would have both spouses affected. The respective proportions would show immediately if person-to-person transmission really was a significant factor in the spread of the disease. In principle, the 'experiment' was easy, and in mid-January 1978 we mentioned it to Dr M. S. Pereira at the Virus Reference Laboratory of the Central Public Health Service. Dr Pereira then kindly informed us that data to this effect existed already. A search of the files showed that there was no significant excess of cases in which both spouses were attacked. While the couples in Dr Pereira's sample were not quite as young as we had envisaged — the average age was thought to be about thirty — person-to-person transmission, if it exists, should have shown up clearly in the data, which it did not.

This was really sufficient to settle the matter, for if person-to-person transmission does not exist, it does not exist. There is a widespread view, however, that since influenza is an exceedingly peculiar disease, anything at all might happen in just one such experiment. We were therefore led to consider what else might be done. By now we had rejected, for the psychological reasons we have mentioned, questionnaires addressed to special groups. The WHO surveillance programme was already covering in depth certain selected sample areas in Britain, and we thought at first that it would be redundant, and likely enough ineffective in view of our limited resources, to attempt any survey of our own. Yet we were constantly reminding ourselves that the opportunity was there, right under our noses as it were, an opportunity which might not present itself again for several years. Moreover, our interests were different from those of the WHO surveillance programme, since our thoughts at that time were concerned with the geographical incidence of the disease on to Britain, and our investigation demanded widespread coverage rather than in-depth surveys over limited areas.

As well as our conversation with Dr Pereira, we also had the benefit of discussions with Dr P. L. Mann in Bath and Dr C. W. L. Howells in Cardiff, and it may well have been a remark in these discussions, that the epidemic in the UK did not look like being a big one, which turned our attention to schools. We argued that because pupils in schools had never been exposed to the new H1 N1, and therefore had no antibody protection against this particular subtype of virus, the attack-rates in schools would be significantly higher than among the older population. Hence it was to schools that we had to look for the most dramatic outbreaks of H1 N1. We do not know whether this argument was correct, or just a lucky mistake, for in the event we did not obtain much in the way of data concerning the influenza subtype(s) responsible for the outbreaks we describe in detail in the next chapter. Possibly the argument was wrong, for by February 1978 the depredations of H1 N1, the so-called Red Flu, were becoming less than those of the variety of H3 N2 first detected in England in 1975 (A/Eng/75), but which the Texans were seeking to appropriate to themselves (A/Texas/77). We have been quite amused to find something of a competition between countries, states and provinces, to become designated as the first point of incidence of each new influenza variety.

The strike of H1 N1 on to the USSR appears to have been severe. Recently we received the data shown in Figure 5.5 from Professor V. M. Zhdanov, Director of the Ivanovsky Institute of Virology. It is worth noting that epidemic peaks were reached almost contemporaneously in the week 19–25 December 1977 for the widely separated cities of Murmansk (68.59N, 33.08E), Kuibyshev (53.10N, 50.10E) and Dyushambe (38.38N, 68.51E), and that the peak at Vladivostok (43.09N, 131.53E) in the week 5–11 December 1977 was not much earlier.

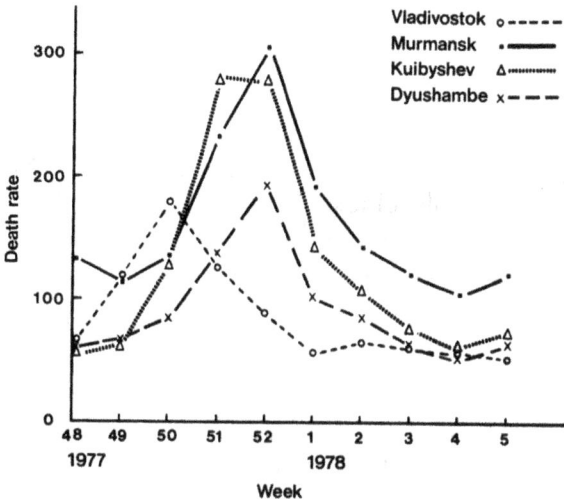

Fig. 5.5.   Death rates from influenza in four widely separated cities in the USSR during the 1977–1978 epidemic (from data supplied by Professor V. M. Zhdanov).

Th question of whether H1 N1 was released in error from a Chinese laboratory sometime in the spring of 1977 was mentioned by Professor Beveridge in a *New Scientist* article published on 23 March 1978. Professor Beveridge says that since the Chinese in the area concerned did not possess H1 N1, this could not be true. For our part, we would add that the evidence to be presented in the next chapter shows that even if someone, the Chinese or otherwise, were to release at ground level an influenza virus in naked form, it would have absolutely no effect.

It was immediately clear that we could not hope to obtain medically attested evidence of every influenza case occurring in a selection of schools distributed throughout Britain, and in this respect any data that we might acquire would be inferior to the data being acquired by the WHO surveillance programme. Yet was this really a serious handicap? Influenza is so well-known to doctors, matrons and nurses, and indeed to the public at large, that misidentifications should be statistically unimportant.

This would be especially so if we confined our investigation to schools which, outside of epidemic outbreaks, had essentially one hundred per cent attendance records. For such schools, all we needed to do was to ensure that an epidemic outbreak of influenza was not confused by the presence of some other disease, for example chicken pox. In practice, we found that this was easy to do, for our sample of schools turned out to be so large that we could simply reject all cases in which matrons and medical officers reported the attack of any disease other than influenza.

While we could not obtain a certificate of guarantee for every reported case of influenza, the use of school pupils as detectors of the influenza virus had formidable advantages. For the most part, class attendance records are meticulously kept in British schools. Absences from class (for schools with otherwise high attendance records) would immediately give us a measure of the attack-rate of the disease. While some pupils and their parents would probably accept a greater measure of discomfort than others, this variation could hardly generate systematic bias, since it would be much the same from class to class and from school to school. The diagnostic criterion of absence from school would therefore be very uniform. It would be quite free of the influence of psychology on diagnosis. Most important of all, none of those involved — victims, matrons and doctors — would know in advance that an 'experiment' was to be performed. We could simply examine attendance records, as well as the records kindly made available to us by matrons and doctors, after the epidemic was over and long forgotten by the victims.

We started this programme with several schools in the Cardiff area. We began tentatively, hoping that something of interest would emerge, and not dreaming that within a few weeks we would have accumulated overwhelming evidence to show that influenza is not a transmitted disease. Influenza descends from the atmosphere, and it does so in an exceedingly patchy distribution. Doubtless there will still be attempts to adapt the concept of a cometary incidence from space, by arguing that the virus gets sucked up from infected persons or animals and is then blown around the troposphere by winds. Because of the susceptibility of the free virus to deactivation we do not think it would be possible to sustain this idea, but it is at least arguable. What is not arguable any more is that influenza passes from person-to-person like a bucket along a line. This idea is now as dead as it should have been from the days of Charles Creighton.

6
Anatomy of an Epidemic

Our decision to investigate the 1978 influenza outbreaks in British schools was lucky from the beginning. Within a day or two of looking through the attendance ledgers of several schools in the Cardiff area we had at last begun to suspect the correctness of the usual claims for the importance of immunity. While a person's immunological history is certainly relevant to whether an attack of influenza turns out to be mild or severe, it is not in our view the primary factor in deciding whether a person succumbs or escapes the disease during an epidemic. In Chapter 3 we have already given one reason why the attack of a respiratory pathogenic virus must be capricious. To reach the Earth and to settle down through the atmosphere, the influenza virus must be embedded within a protective matrix, probably of organic material, perhaps even consisting of a bacterium or other living cell. When such an embedded virus is breathed, there is the critical issue of whether the virus becomes free while the larger host particle remains within the respiratory tract. The drinking of a cup or glass of liquid may wash the particle down into the stomach, and it may well be more or less random events of this kind that decide the apparently capricious nature of attacks of influenza and of the common cold. This is why there are so many cases in which one spouse contracts influenza and the other escapes. The discriminations of the disease are not to be explained by variations of immunity. Indeed to a first approximation (for any reasonably coherent community) all people are to be taken as equally susceptible. In our view the effects of immunity appear only at second order.

We soon saw from the school attendance records that pupils across the age-range of a particular school were much more similar to each other in their response to the influenza epidemic than they were to pupils in other schools. Since we could not believe that pupils in different schools were inherently different from each other, this meant that some other factor had to be controlling the situation, which we attributed immediately to the patchy incidence of the influenza virus on to the Cardiff area.

The geographical positions of the schools in question are shown in Figure 6.1, with additional details of pupil numbers given in Table 6.1. Figure 6.2 gives a comparison of 'excess absences' during the influenza epidemic between the whole of Howell's School and the youngest girls in the first two forms. To obtain 'excess absences' we subtracted from the actual absences the much smaller absences — about three per cent — that occurred over periods adjacent to, but well clear of, the epidemic. Figure 6.3 compares school totals for Howell's with those for Llanishen High and St Cyres.

Here was indisputable evidence to show that geographical location was of far greater importance than the age variability of pupils, a conclusion which emerged at a later stage of our investigation

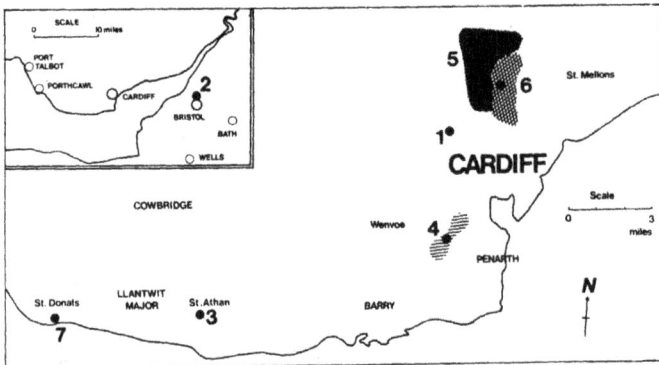

Fig. 6.1. Locations of West Country schools included in our preliminary study. Hatched zones represent catchment areas where known. Numbers refer to Howell's (1), Clifton (2), Balfour House (3), St Cyres (4), Llanishen High (5), Cardiff High (6) and Atlantic College (7).

Table 6.1.

School	No. of Day-Pupils	No. of Boarders	Location	Catchment Area
1. Howell's (girls)	454	96	Llandaff, about 3 miles West of Cardiff Centre	Day-pupils: large
2. Clifton (boys)	256	421	Clifton Downs, Bristol	Day-pupils large
3. Balfour House (boys)	223	—	St Athan, about 12 miles West of Cardiff Centre on coast	Large
4. St Cyres (mixed)	316	—	Dinas Powis, about 5 miles South-West of Cardiff Centre	Very small
5. Llanishen High (mixed)	About 1,400	—	Llanishen, about 3 miles North of Cardiff Centre	Small
6. Cardiff High (mixed)	About 1,700	—	Cardiff Centre	Small

in an overwhelming form. Visits to actual classrooms convinced us that even the firmest adherent to the concept of person-to-person transmission could not argue for there being much of a difference in the spacing of desks from one school to another. Nor could it be argued that there is much difference in the play habits in the different schools, as for instance in the extent to which pupils whisper, talk or huddle together. Giving the person-to-person transmission hypothesis the fairest possible run for its money, we could see no way to interpret the evidence of Figures 6.2 and 6.3 satisfactorily in terms of this hypothesis. Person-to-person transmission should have produced closely similar patterns, but the patterns were not similar.

Next we attempted to test the possibility that there might be a systematic difference between country schools and city-centre schools. Rising air over cities might help to ward off an infalling pathogen. Pollutants in the atmosphere over cities might coat particles, so providing some measure of protection for city centres. On the other hand if such particles once entered a city, they could well blow around for quite a long time, whereas virus embedded in an organic capsule would tend to become stuck firmly to leaves and to grass whenever it fell in the countryside, and so would not readily be stirred up into the air again by the wind. There were ample reasons therefore to suspect that cities and countryside might be different.

At first we thought these expectations could be subject to a quick test, but it was only much later that we were in fact able to obtain real weight of evidence for city-centre schools. The problem was the high endemic truancy with which city-centre state schools are afflicted. We did find one school, Cardiff High, not too far from the city centre, at which the normal attendance record was high enough for an interesting hint to be forthcoming. The excess absences for Cardiff High are shown in Figure 6.4, together with those of Balfour House and Clifton College. Whereas the latter followed patterns similar to those we have seen in Figure 6.3, the situation for Cardiff High was evidently different. It is plain to be seen that the influenza virus makes no distinction as to the culture

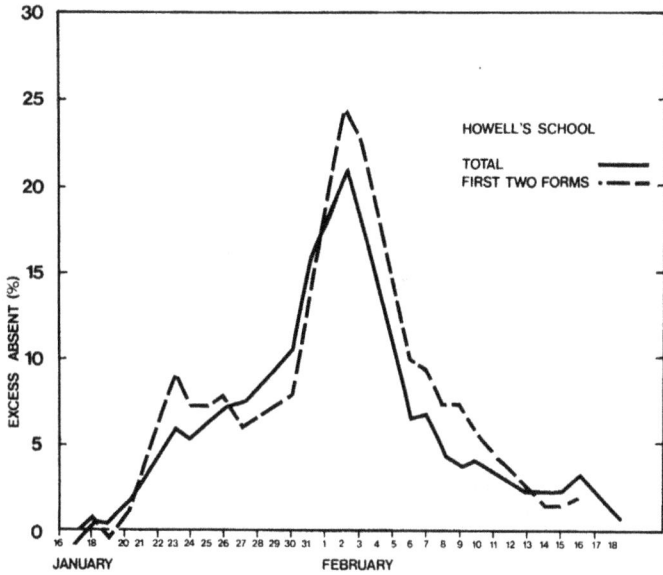

Fig. 6.2. Excess absences (per cent) above normal for Howell's School. The two curves show absences for whole school and for pupils in the first two forms only.

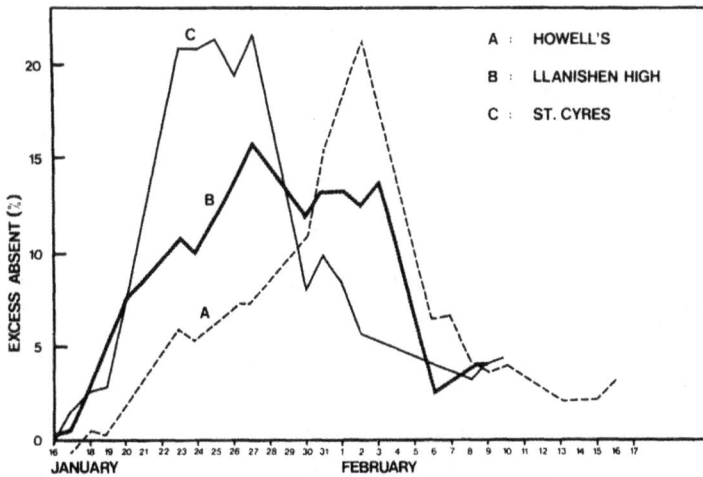

Fig. 6.3. Excess total absences (per cent) above normal for Howell's, Llanishen High and St Cyres Dinas Powis.

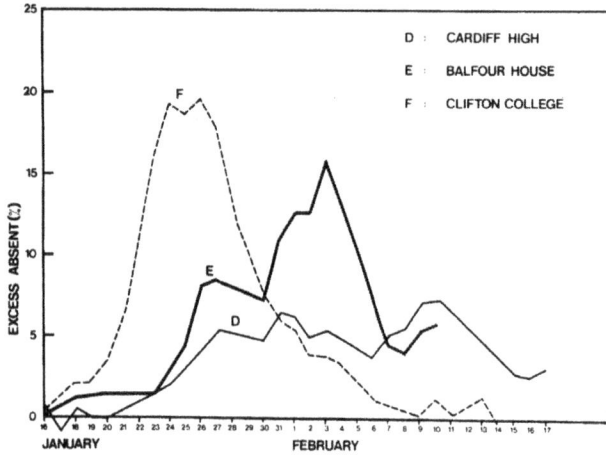

Fig. 6.4. Excess total absences (per cent) above normal for Cardiff High, Balfour House and Clifton College.

or the economic fortunes of those whom it attacks. The situation for St Cyres, a Welsh country state school, was almost identical with that of Clifton College, a fee-paying independent English school. These two schools must have been hit contemporaneously by almost identical pathogenic patches of virus.

It will be noticed that while seven schools are marked in Figure 6.1, only six of them appear in Table 6.1 and in Figures 6.2 to 6.4. The seventh school is St Donat's. It was a further piece of good fortune that we encountered such a very exceptional case early in our investigation. This sixth-form school has many unique features. It is built around the fourteenth-century St Donat's Castle and is situated on an exposed cliff overlooking St Donat's Bay. The nearest town is Llantwit Major. The school draws students from all parts of the world who wish to qualify for admission to British and American universities. It is financed by international educational organisations and has its own recreational, residential and academic facilities. There are 343 students between the ages of 16 and 19, all in residence, in 8 houses scattered on the campus. During the period 13 February–3 March, the school suffered an attack of acute upper respiratory disease. No class attendance records are kept, but the sister in charge of the Medical Centre gave us access to her records of case admissions to the school infirmary. All forty-eight recorded cases of influenza were found to be febrile, the duration of acute illness being four to five days.

From our point of view the importance of the school lay in the facilities of the dormitories which were built in the past decade. Because of high modern building costs there was no possibility of constructing large rooms with high ceilings such as could afforded in the more spacious days when most other independent schools were built. The dormitories were built functionally, and with a few exceptions they were all of the same sleeping capacity, with four pupils to a dormitory. The situation was essentially the same as it would have been for 85 dormitories, each with 4 persons to it.

At St Donat's the pupils work, eat and play communally, going to the dormitories only to sleep. Much time is spent out-of-doors, when according to our point of view pupils would be more at risk than indoors. If we were correct in our belief that most of the forty-eight cases would have been contracted out-of-doors, and if we were also correct in thinking that there could be no subsequent person-to-person transmission of the disease, the forty-eight cases would inevitably be randomly distributed with respect to the dormitories. If, on the other hand, person-to-person transmission had taken place, then regardless of where the disease had been caught there would be non-random clusterings of cases within the dormitories. The only situation in which we ourselves would expect non-random clustering would be if the influenza had been contracted within the actual dormitories themselves, but because of the exceptional situation at St Donat's there was a good chance that this had not been so.

The sister, Miss Stanley, kindly assisted us in sorting the forty-eight cases into the dormitories where they had occurred, and as the work proceeded she became more and more astonished to find how many of the dormitories had only a single victim. If one were to distribute 48 apples randomly into 85 boxes, the most likely distribution would be 1 box with 3 apples, 7 boxes with 2 apples, 31 boxes with 1 apple, and the rest with nothing, the proportions of the apple-containing boxes being given approximately by the binomial terms

$$1:\frac{1}{2!}\times\frac{47}{84}:\frac{1}{3!}\times\frac{47\cdot46}{84^2}.$$

At St Donat's there was 1 dormitory with 3 victims, 5 dormitories with 2 victims, 35 dormitories with 1 victim, and the rest with nothing. This meant that there was slightly less clustering than we would expect for a typical random allotment, although not by an amount that we considered to be significant.

Up to this point we had found plenty of evidence against the person-to-person transmission of influenza. Yet even so, we had hesitated to be as forthright as Charles Creighton in maintaining that person-to-person transmission does not occur. Whereas one needs only the flimsiest evidence to hold a popular point of view, it is necessary to have much solid evidence to oppose the popular view, or at any rate to do so in a relaxed state of mind. From the moment we saw the St Donat's data, we had our relaxed frame of mind. Here was a situation that could hardly have been improved upon in a planned experiment. From that moment onwards we knew that influenza is not a transmitted disease.

It was also lucky that we had chosen to look at the dormitory situation at St Donat's ahead of that for Howell's, since the latter turned out to be more complex, but nevertheless just as remarkable. Fortified now by what we had learned at St Donat's, we turned to unravelling the Howell's situation. Luckily again, Miss Morgan, the sister at Howell's, was able to supply us not only with diagrams of the dormitories and with the positions of the beds occupied by the thirty-six boarders who had succumbed during the epidemic, but also with the order in which the victims had presented themselves for treatment. The data are shown in a schematic way in Figure 6.5, where we have stylised the shapes of the dormitories (which varied considerably from one dormitory to another) and have marked the victims in a way that omits details of their actual positions, which were much more mixed up than our figure suggests — the victims and those who escaped were not in the neat orderly arrangement that might perhaps be suggested by the figure. Pupils marked H in the figure live comparatively near the school and succumbed to the virus during the weekend at home.

The numbers marked in Figure 6.5 refer to sequential order in contracting the disease, so that 18 means the 18th victim to report the onset of illness. Because of the sharpness of the main peak of the epidemic at Howell's (see Figure 6.1) we were informed that all numbers after 10 should be considered as essentially contemporaneous. The victims were streaming into the school sick bay within a short time of each other, so that there was no possibility of one of them having infected another. They were simultaneous strikes of the influenza virus.

There were evidently many examples of simultaneous strikes. Going through the dormitories from top left of Figure 6.5 to bottom right, and excluding the 4 H victims, we have the following contemporaneous groupings (10, 25, 31), (14, 24), (11, 12), (21, 22), (13, 15, 19), (28, 29), (26, 27). Thus 16 of the 32 victims were involved in simultaneous strikes. We have no means of knowing whether these strikes occurred in the houses or in the dormitories, nor do we know whether some of the groupings were of particular friends who went everywhere around the school together. We were tempted to seek the latter information but decided that our enquiry should not involve itself in the personal lives of the pupils of this or any other school. Conceivably we might have gained from seeking such information in particular cases, but in the long run we would inevitably have introduced psychological bias into the results.

Is there any support for person-to-person transmission in the data of Figure 6.5? Certainly not from groupings like (13, 15, 19) which were contemporaneous, but what of the particular dormitory at top left with victims 1, 2, 4, 6? Did victim 1 infect the others, or was this dormitory the first to be hit by a strike of the virus on to Hazelwood from outside of the house itself? To decide this question, we noted that if transmission had occurred, there would be an excess of victims in the larger dormitories. But if there was not person-to-person transmission then the chance of contracting the disease would be much the same, irrespective of the sizes of

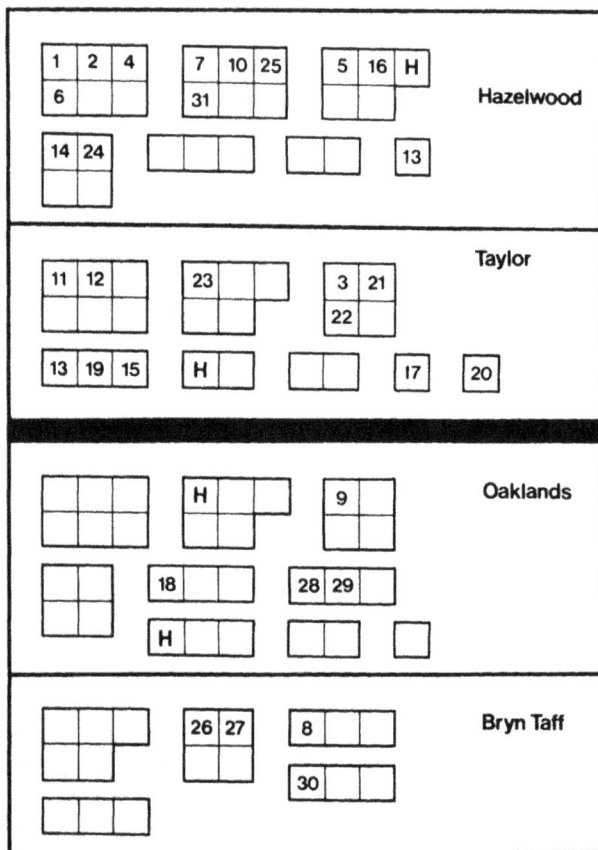

Fig. 6.5. Schematic plan of dormitories at Howell's for four houses: Hazelwood, Taylor, Oaklands and Bryn Taff. Boxes represent rooms, compartments within boxes are occupied beds. Numbers show order of victims reporting to the school nurse. H stands for a week-day boarder who had influenza over the weekend.

the dormitories, in which case the larger dormitories would simply have numbers of victims in proportion to the numbers of their beds. Table 6.2 shows the result of making this test.

For the houses Hazelwood and Taylor considered together, there were 26 victims from a total of 51 pupils, giving an attack-rate of $26/51 = 0.51$. The averages in the third column of the

Table 6.2. Test of person-to-person transmission hypothesis in dormitories at Howell's School.

No. of beds in dormitory	No. of such dormitories in Hazelwood and Taylor	Average no. of victims expected in such dormitories if assigned cases were distributed randomly	Actual no. of cases
6	3	9.18	10
5	2	5.10	4
4	2	4.08	5
3	2	3.06	3

2 ⎫
  ⎬
1 ⎭
	3 ⎫
	  ⎬
	3 ⎭
		3.06 ⎫
		        ⎬ 4.59
		1.53 ⎭
			1 ⎫
			  ⎬ 4
			3 ⎭

table are obtained by multiplying this attack-rate by the numbers of beds contained in dormitories of various sizes. Thus for 6-bed dormitories there were 18 beds in three such dormitories, and $18 \times 0.51 = 9.18$. Comparisons with actual numbers of victims are all close, except when the number of beds involved becomes small for the 1-bed and 2-bed dormitories. These latter fluctuations also become small, however, when the 1-bed and 2-bed dormitories are totalled together (thereby reducing the statistical scatter of the numbers). This evidence therefore supported our findings at St Donat's. There was no person-to-person transmission of the disease, even though in this case the virus would appear to have struck at the houses themselves.

The houses in Figure 6.5 fall into two pairs, Hazelwood and Taylor, with a total of 26 victims out of 51 pupils, and Oaklands and Bryn Taff, with only 10 victims out of 49 pupils. Was this difference a random effect, or was the difference to be taken as a real variation of the strike of the virus on the two pairs of houses? Figure 6.6 shows the geographical location of the houses, and

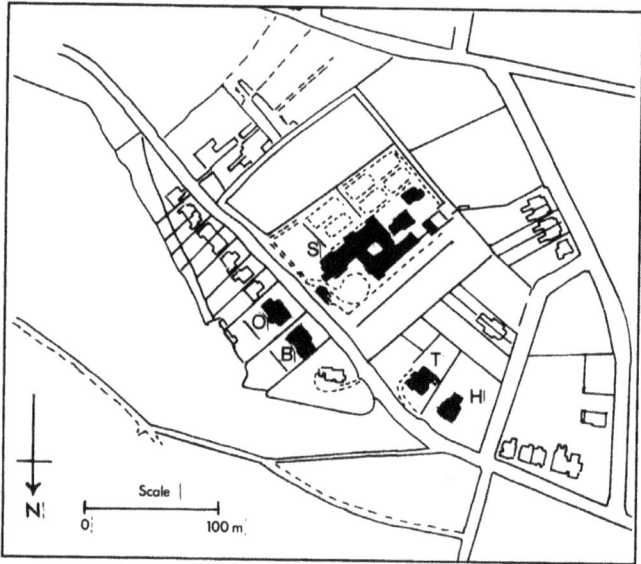

Fig. 6.6. Map of area around Howell's School — S refers to main School; O refers to Oaklands House; B refers to Bryn Taff House; T refers to Taylor House; H refers to Hazelwood House.

sure enough they are positioned in two pairs, and the two pairs are indeed Hazelwood–Taylor and Oaklands–Bryn Taff. Yet the pairs are a mere hundred yards apart, and could the virus really be patchy on so fine a scale? We had been prepared for patchiness on the scale of the whole of Cardiff, a scale of several miles, but not on a scale as small as this. But could this difference be a mere random effect? So what was the chance, if one were to make a random allotment of 36 apples into two essentially equal boxes, of finding that 26 apples had gone into one of the boxes and only 10 into the other box? The answer was a chance of about 1 in 140. And if one were to include all the still more unequal possibilities, such as 27 apples going into one box and only 9 into the other, 28 into one box and 8 into the other, and so on, the chance of any one of these unusual distributions turning up would be about 1 in 100. The chance was small enough to make us suspect that we had come on a real effect, not a mere statistical fluctuation, but perhaps not small enough to force us to this conclusion, since the conclusion was far too remarkable to be accepted lightly. Evidently the matter needed further investigation, and for this we had to look to schools outside the Cardiff area. Eventually we were to receive a veritable torrent of information showing that our first suspicions derived from the Howell's data were indeed correct. The incidence of the influenza virus is patchy on a scale of a hundred yards, and probably on a scale even less than this. We shall come to the explanation of this remarkable fact at the end of this chapter.

The time was now mid-March 1978. Epidemic attacks of influenza in schools were dying away, and within a few weeks memories would fade, so that the precise meaning of entries in notebooks and ledgers would become difficult to recover. A great quantity of precious information would be gone, long before we ourselves could do anything about collecting it in person. The best that might be done in a personal way would be to double the amount of information we had obtained already, and this would be quite insufficient to answer the question that was uppermost in our minds at that time. Had there been broad meteorological patterns of incidence of the virus? How did Charles Creighton's spreading 'miasma' over the land really look?

To answer these questions, it would evidently be necessary to send out a questionnaire to a large number of schools. The problem with a questionnaire was that it would need to be simple. We ourselves have received many complex questionnaires sent out by scientific committees and we well know the confusion and irritation they cause. To be feasible a questionnaire would need to be confined to one side of a single sheet (the irritation begins when you turn over and find more questions on the other side). On one side of a single sheet we were able to ask for total school absences from classes over a three-week period, centred around the epidemic peak, listed separately for day-pupils and boarders (in the event that a school had both day-pupils and boarders and in the event of course that a school actually experienced an epidemic). We also asked that the total number of victims be given, again separately for day-pupils and boarders. Unfortunately this particular question was not unambiguously worded and only about a half of the replies interpreted it in the way we had intended.

There was clearly no hope of dealing through a questionnaire with the more complex issues of dormitories and houses. Because every school would have its own individual features (St Donat's and Howell's had been very different) no uniform set of questions would suffice, even if the involved nature of such an enquiry would have been tolerated. What we did was to ask if schools had data for houses, without actually asking for the data, so that at this stage we were only asking for a simple yes-or-no answer. Through this easily-answered last question we would obtain a short-list of schools to which further more detailed enquiries might be added. This, at any rate, was our idea at that point.

There were two reasons for sending out the questionnaire only to independent schools. These were the schools that would have interesting dormitory and house-distribution data, and these would be the schools that would be free from the city truancy problem of state schools. We wrote a report of our findings, covered here by Figures 6.1 to 6.6, and sent the report out with a questionnaire to more than 500 independent schools. Within a few weeks we had received a large number of replies, weighted obviously towards the schools that had suffered epidemic attacks, although some fifty schools replied that they had experienced no attack. Our favourite negative reply came from a headmistress who wrote: 'I am delighted to say that we had no epidemic of influenza. This school rarely, if ever, has epidemics. I think we are too high on a hill.' The headmistress' opinion about being high on a hill could be well-founded for we had a reply from Rydal School in North Wales with the following interesting details. The senior school is in nine houses sited on the slopes of a hill, while the junior school is in woodland at the very top of the hill. The senior school had 109 victims out of a total of 289 pupils, while the junior school had zero victims out of a total of 121 pupils. Since this was not a quarantine situation — there was contact between the two schools — the evidence for an advantageous connection with the hill top seems overwhelming. A few of the negative replies attributed their escape to vaccination programmes, and one or two medical officers implied that if others had adopted such programmes there would have been no influenza. If these medical officers had seen the scathing comments from other schools which had used the same vaccines, but which had nevertheless suffered exceedingly high attack-rates of the disease, they would perhaps have been less complacent. The information concerning vaccination programmes was unsolicited by us, and so it may well have had psychological bias.

Charles Creighton was not correct in detail in his thinking of a cloud of disease spreading over the land. We soon saw that the situation was far more complex than this. Nor does the disease spread like a bucket handed along a line of people, as it would tend to do through person-to-person transmission. It jumps about all over the place. We shall come to a discussion of the meteorology of this 'jumping-about' at the end of the present chapter. Generally speaking, the smaller units of area that one examines the more apparently capricious is the incidence of the disease. Table 6.3 which gives day-by-day absence of boarders at Headington School, Oxford, according to houses, illustrates this point.

Plainly, Latimer House was drastically hit at some time around 3 February (allowing three days for incubation), whereas the other four houses escaped with much lighter blows.

Attack-rates on day-pupils tend to be smoothed over the whole catchment area of a school, thereby giving a clearer indication than boarders of the broad features of the incidence of the disease on to the whole country. We had 72 schools with adequate numbers of day-pupils for the attack-rates on them to be well determined. These we divided into 4 categories: 0–25 per cent attack-rates; 25–50 per cent; 50–75 per cent; and 75–100 per cent. The numbers of schools in these categories respectively were 21, 30, 18, 3.

Isolated communities in polar regions or on mid-oceanic islands do not have an entire monopoly on exceedingly high attack-rates, as the Brighton experience (98 per cent) showed. The lowest category of 0–25 per cent was dominant either along the south coast from Cornwall to Sussex, or over the Greater London area. The 25–50 per cent category had a rather smooth distribution throughout the

Table 6.3. Class-absences of boarders at Headington School, Oxford classified according to houses.

House	*Davenport* (34 pupils)	*Hillstow* (63 pupils)	*Latimer* (46 pupils)	*Napier* (42 pupils)	*Celia Marsh* (44 pupils)
Date					
30 Jan	1	7	2	6	8
31	5	10	3	7	6
1 Feb	3	12	1	6	4
2	6	10	2	3	5
3	7	8	6	3	4
6	3	4	26	9	5
7	1	4	26	6	3
8	2	4	22	4	3
9	1	1	25	3	3
10	2	1	20	5	3
13	0	4	6	0	0
14	0	2	3	2	1
15	0	3	1	2	0
16	0	2	0	2	1
17	0	2	2	2	0

whole country, whereas the 50–75 per cent category was dominant over a great arc which begins in the north-east at Ely, goes west to Northampton and then turns south to Oxford and Reading. Turning now back towards the east, the arc continues well south of London through Godalming and Horsham, ending at Maidstone in Kent. Along the arc were thirteen schools. Nowhere over Greater London was there an attack-rate above 35 per cent. This was the answer to our question about the shielding effect of cities. When the attack-rates are plotted in detail on a wall map (or see

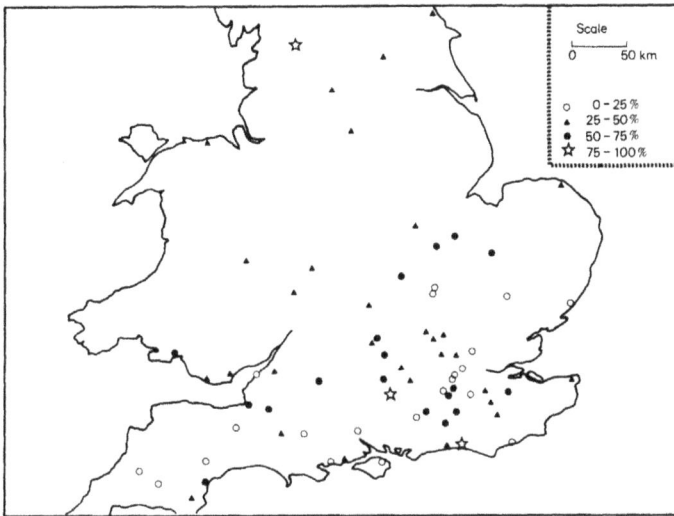

Fig. 6.7. Distribution of day-pupil attack rates during the 1978 influenza epidemic in England and Wales.

Figure 6.7) the low values over London stand out immediately, as does the great arc described above.

At this point, we mention a device we used to interpret some of the data. About half of the replies gave us both class absences and total numbers of victims. The remainder gave us only class absences, and for these we could not determine attack-rates directly. In some cases where critical issues were concerned we telephoned the schools in question asking for total numbers, but for the rest we proceeded in the following way. From the half for which we had complete data, by dividing total class absences by numbers of victims we found that on the average each victim was absent from classes for close to five days. We then took five days to be the number of days for which victims in the other half had been absent from classes. In short, dividing total class absences by five gave us the number of victims in the cases where this information was not contained directly in the replies. The procedure could have introduced a modest error in the attack-rates deduced for particular schools, but it cannot have introduced systematic bias.

ATTACK-RATES

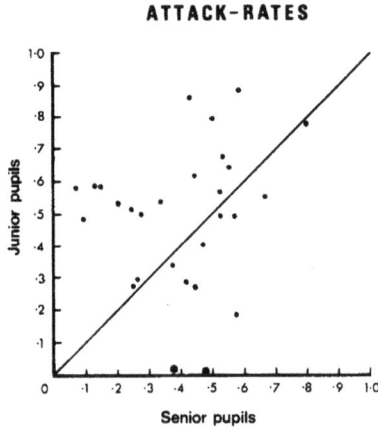

Fig. 6.8. Correlation of attack-rates for Junior and Senior pupils (Junior 5 to 13: Senior from 14).

The larger filled circles represent schools where the Junior pupils have been virtually unscathed. The eye can detect about 10 per cent in the data towards a higher attack rate on Juniors. This is a fluctuation at about one standard deviation which would arise at random with 30 per cent probability, or the bias could be due to a 10 per cent increased susceptibility of Juniors to attack by the influenza virus; or it could be due to the greater solicitude which parents and school authorities generally have for Juniors. More data will be required to decide between these three possibilities.

  We had ample confirmation of the difference between urban schools and country schools, the city schools with broad flat distributions and the country schools with sudden sharp peaks, just as we had found for the Cardiff area. But while in our own survey we had not found much difference in the attack-rates on the youngest and oldest pupils, we now found considerable differences for those schools which reported attack-rates on both preparatory schools and senior schools. Nevertheless, when we plotted the numbers on the correlation diagram of Figure 6.8 we found that the points for this limited sample of schools were scattered about a line of 45° slope, indicating that any difference of susceptibility between the younger and older pupils was really as unimportant as we ourselves had found it to be. Some other much more important factor was evidently involved in producing the scatter of points in Figure 6.8. In our own survey, all pupils had occupied the same buildings. Here seniors and juniors were usually occupying different buildings. At The King's School, Ely, the situation was much the same as in our own survey, and at The King's School the attack-rates were: Senior day pupils, 57 per cent; Junior day pupils, 56 per cent; Senior boarden, 56 per cent; Junior boarden, 57 per cent. This was another hint of how crucially important buildings can be in their effect on influenza attack-rates, a conclusion that was eventually to be driven home to us with overwhelming force.

We also found no significant difference of susceptibility between day pupils and boarders. For individual schools there were often marked differences, which we expected to find because day pupils occupy the whole catchment area of a school in the hours between about 5.00 p.m. and 9.00 a.m. (i.e. for two-thirds of the time), whereas boarders remain at the particular location of the school. But when the attack-rates were plotted on a correlation diagram, as in Figure 6.9 with each point representing an individual school, no significant difference remained. It so happened that many of the

ATTACK-RATES

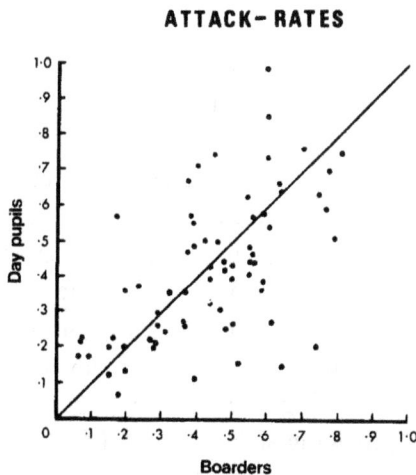

Fig. 6.9. Correlation of attack rates for Day pupils and Boarders in schools which had a mixture of both.

schools gave us an estimate of their absentee rate for day pupils, which ran typically at about 3 per cent. We reduced the influenza attack-rates on day pupils to allow for this effect, but made no corresponding adjustment for boarders. Since it is unlikely that boarders really have a 100 per cent attendance at classes outside of an influenza epidemic, there must be a slight bias in our analysis towards overweighting the attack-rate on boarders, an overweighting that can perhaps just be detected in Figure 6.9.

We had scarcely dared hope that our simple questionnaire would provide the more complex information necessary for following up the investigations of dormitories and school houses that we had begun at Howell's and St Donat's. Fortunately, however, such data were indeed forthcoming from about thirty of the schools, where medical officers and school matrons went to the trouble to send to us a great deal of interesting data, some of which we have still not analysed in the depth which they deserve. It is matter for regret that space does not allow us here to do more than pick out a few of the highlights from this rich body of material. Returning for a moment to the matter of questionnaires, a glance at these particular replies shows that we had again been lucky in not attempting to define in advance what points would be of importance. Each school had its own individual features, and many had peculiar experiences that we could not have foreseen. There would have been no possibility of designing a grandiose questionnaire bringing all this information to light.

Here we shall confine the discussion of these special replies to one topic, the influence of buildings on influence attack-rates. As a prelude to the discussion, it will be useful to mention a few ideas in the theory of probability. To illustrate the calculation of what is called the 'standard deviation', we can consider the experiment of tossing a penny n times. The standard deviation for this experiment is obtained by taking the square root of $np(p-1)$, with p the probability of throwing a head, and $(1-p)$ the probability of throwing a tail. It is usual to think of a penny as being unbiased, by which one means that throwing a head or tail is equally likely, so that $p = 0.5$. If we chose to toss a penny 64 times, then

$np(1-p) = 16$, and the square root of this is 4. Thus 4 is the standard deviation for the experiment of tossing an unbiased penny 64 times.

If one were actually to toss a penny 64 times, it would be rather unlikely for the number of heads to be 32. If one did the experiment several times, sometimes the number would be more than 32, and sometimes less than 32, with 32 appearing as the average result of many such experiments. The deviation from 32 in a particular experiment is known as the fluctuation in that experiment, and fluctuations are measured in terms of the standard deviation. Thus 28 heads in an experiment would be one standard deviation below the average, and 36 heads would be one standard deviation above the average, while 24 heads or 40 heads would be fluctuations of two standard deviations, and so on.

Now we can ask what the chances are for fluctuations of various amounts to turn up. The situation for the experiment of tossing a penny 64 times is shown in Table 6.4. The table shows that in about one such experiment in three, the number of heads obtained would turn out either to be less than 28 or more than 36 (i.e. outside the range 28 to 36). However, one would need to do the experiment about 1000 million times before the number of heads would be less than 8 or more than 56. If in practice, one were to obtain less than 8 or more than 56 heads then it would be wise to suspect that the penny was biased. Detection of bias in what is supposed to be a random situation is indeed one of the main purposes of this kind of fluctuation analysis, as for instance detection of bias in the spin of a roulette wheel.

Table 6.4 has a value far beyond the experiment of tossing a penny 64 times. If we forget this experiment and imagine the middle column of the table removed, the first and third columns can be applied to any yes-or-no situation in which we know the probability of a 'yes' answer. In our consideration of the way that 36 victims at Howell's fell into the house pairs Hazelwood–Taylor and Oaklands–Bryn Taff, we considered 36 apples being allotted randomly into two equal boxes, say A and B. The possibility of each apple going in one of the boxes, say A, is 1/2. We take this to

Table 6.4. Fluctuations in the number of 'heads' obtained in the experiment of tossing penny 64 times.

Fluctuation more than:	Result outside the range:		Chance of happening:
1 standard deviation	28 to 36	about	1 in 3
2 standard deviations	24 to 40	"	1 in 22
3 standard deviations	20 to 44	"	1 in 370
4 standard deviations	16 to 48	"	1 in 16,000
5 standard deviations	12 to 52	"	1 in 2 million
6 standard deviations	8 to 56	"	1 in 1000 million

be our 'yes' answer, so that $p = 1/2$, just as in the tossing of a penny. For 36 such allotments we have $n = 36$, and the standard deviation $\sqrt{np(1-p)}$ in 3 exactly. The average np is 18. In the actual experience of the influenza epidemic at Howell's. Hazelwood–Taylor had 26 victims, which exceeded the average by 8, a difference of $8/3 = 2.67$ standard deviations. Table. 6.4 shows that the chance of a fluctuation as large as this was about 1 in 100, as we stated above.

We proceeded in an exactly similar way for the results which we received in answer to our questionnaire. We had many cases in which the fluctuations of the actual numbers of victims exceeded three standard deviations, which is usually taken as the breakpoint at which one decides that the situation has bias: the allotments of victims were not random. This inevitably implied that the school houses must somehow have been involved in determining numbers of victims, either through their geographical locations (for instance by being on top of a hill) or in some other way (for instance by somebody opening a window and so admitting the virus at a crucial moment).

As a first example, the two larger houses at St Mary's, Calne, have 55 and 57 boarders, and the numbers of victims in them were 35 and 2, respectively. With the slight approximation of taking the houses to be equal one has the same problem as at Howell's, but with 37 victims instead of 36. If we also neglect this small difference, the standard deviation would again be 3 and the average expectation would again be 18 victims in each house. The fluctuation now, however, is about 16, more than 5 standard deviations, with a chance of happening at random according to Table 6.4 of less than 1 in 2 million. The indication of bias — in other words, of the house buildings being involved — was therefore much stronger at St Mary's than it had been at Howell's.

The most extreme fluctuations were at Eton College, Windsor. Figure 6.10 shows our calculated numbers of standard deviations for each of the twenty-five houses at Eton. Downward fluctuations indicate that numbers of victims were less than expected averages, and upwards fluctuations were for excesses above the averages, which were calculated in the following way. For the whole school there were 441 victims among 1248 pupils, for an attack-rate of $411/1248 = 0.35$. The expected average for a house was obtained simply by multiplying the number of pupils in the house by 0.35. Thus for College House with 70 pupils, the expected average of victims was $70 \times 0.35 = 25$ approximately. The actual number of victims in College House was 1, for a fluctuation of about 24 which amounted to about 6 standard deviations, with a chance of happening (if College House itself had nothing to do with it) of about 1 in 1000 million. With as many as twenty-five houses at Eton we would have thought it just as peculiar if any one of the others had shown a fluctuation of 6 standard deviations. So more properly we should say that the chance against such a fluctuation (again if the houses themselves were not involved) was 1 in 40 million. But there are at least four other houses also with large fluctuations, RHP, MAN, MFW and CAI. If these are taken together with College House, the chance of the Eton situation being 'unbiased' is as little as 1 in 100,000,000,000,000,000. That is to say, one would need to have 100,000,000,000,000,000 epidemics of comparable severity at Eton before a random fluctuation as large as that of Figure 6.10 would occur.

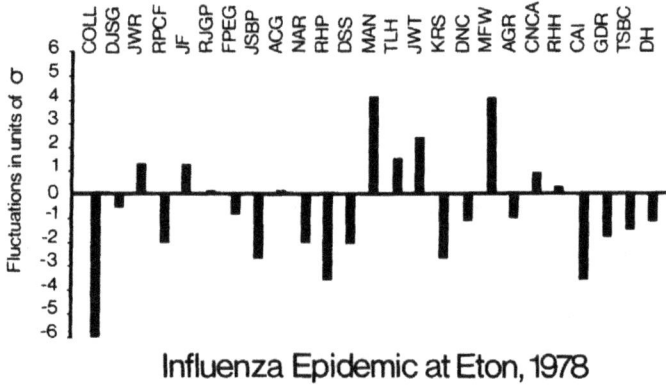

Influenza Epidemic at Eton, 1978

Fig. 6.10. Fluctuations from expected mean numbers of victims in several houses at Eton College. Fluctuations are expressed in terms of standard deviation (0).

When we communicated this result to Dr J. Briscoe, the Medical Officer at Eton, he kindly sent us comparable information for the epidemic years of 1974 and 1976. They showed just the same influence of the school buildings. Thus the chance against the 1974 situation being a random happening was 1 in 100 million, and the chance against the 1976 situation was about 1 in 10,000,000,000,000,000, almost the same as in 1978. This evidence may be considered as entirely decisive in establishing that particular buildings play a critical role in the determination of influenza attack-rates. There was some indication that particular buildings tended to have systematically high or systematically low attack-rates from one epidemic to another (we had a similar indication from St Mary's, Calne), but there was no firm rule to this effect. Nor do we think there should necessarily be such a rule. It could be a matter of chance whether the virus is admitted to one building or to another at a critical moment. On the other hand, once the virus was admitted there could be systematic differences from one building to another, depending on the length of time for which the virus was permitted to remain viable. For example, buildings with many exposed hot surfaces, or with ducted hot-air heating systems, might be expected to destroy the virus more quickly than other buildings.

The Eton results were another blow for the person-to-person transmission hypothesis. Some of the houses which showed very different attack-rates nevertheless have communal eating facilities. And College House could not have remained essentially unscathed if there had been transmission in school classes. The phenomenon of one or more houses escaping unscathed occurred also in the earlier epidemics at Eton, as it did at St Mary's, Calne, and also at about half a dozen other schools. None of this would be possible if there were appreciable transmission of the disease.

Queen Margaret's, York sent us attack-rates according to school classes. We had not thought to make any such enquiry because it had not occurred to us that the incidence of the influenza virus could be patchy on a scale as small as a classroom (the hundred-yard scale at Howell's had seemed astonishingly small). Yet if we assume an unbiased situation (in this case that the classrooms were not involved) the fluctuations in standard deviations for the six most senior forms at Queen Margaret's would be 0.75, 4.18, 3.58, 2.77, 0.05, 2.17, far too large for the assumption of an unbiased situation to be sustained. So the classrooms were involved at Queen Margaret's, demanding a very fine-scale patchiness for the virus.

This sets the meteorological problem. How can a pathogen incident from space on the Earth's upper atmosphere, with a distribution that must surely be of far larger scale in its variations than the dimensions of a school, or a town, and probably even than a whole country or continent, nevertheless end up at ground level in the detailed patchy form that we were now finding? Pathogenic particles of large size, greater in diameter than about five microns (five parts in ten thousandth of a centimetre), would fall through the stratosphere in a few months, and would be washed down through the troposphere in at most a few weeks (see Appendix 2). There would be no particular patchiness in this smooth incidence, so that the fall to ground level of such comparatively large particles would be widespread on an international scale.

For smaller particles, however, the quickest way down through the lower stratosphere would be through storm activity, which would have distinctive local features. Nevertheless, these features would still be much larger than the environs of a school. They would be on the scale of the track of a storm, more like the great arc that we described around London for schools with high attack-rates (50–75 per cent). Storms can bring down particles in two ways: for particles less than five millionths of a centimetre through electrical effects, and for particles in the general visual range (fifty millionths of a centimetre) through eddies of air extending between the troposphere and the stratosphere.

The first step in producing detailed local patterns in the fall of small particles is therefore through storm activity, which brings the particles into the upper troposphere, where they serve as nuclei in the formation of raindrops. This leads to patchiness on the scale of a rain formation, which may be a big cumulus cloud, but more likely for the UK, especially in winter, it would be a frontal disturbance, bigger than a single cumulus cloud.

Next, we notice that it is hardly likely that a respiratory pathogen enclosed in drops of rain will do us much harm. We are not given to snuffling large droplets up into the nose, although for virus which could enter through the cornea of the eye the situation would be different — it has been suggested that measles can enter the body in this way. We therefore have an apparent contradiction. Rain is needed to bring a pathogen down from the upper troposphere, and yet enclosed in raindrops the pathogen is likely to fall on to the ground and to be simply washed away in streams and rivers, or down the gutters in towns and cities. There is one condition, however, that renders an apparently safe situation unsafe, namely the evaporation of droplets that have fallen only part way from the upper atmosphere. Evaporation occurs on stormy days, often during frontal conditions, when the skies suddenly (and it seems miraculously) clear themselves and we find ourselves looking through to the blue sky above. This is the dangerous condition, for it releases the pathogenic particles from their enclosing raindrops. In this way the particles are brought down into the lower atmosphere, but still hundreds or even thousands of feet above our heads. The last step occurs when the lower air is stirred up by locally generated turbulence. It is this final turbulence that carries the virus, by a kind of tumbling motion of the air, down to ground level where we may breathe it.

Strong winds favour the generation of turbulence, although on their own they are by no means sufficient. A wind can blow over a smooth level plane or over the ocean without the generation of turbulence, but a wind blowing over an irregular surface becomes turbulent if it is strong enough. For wind blowing over the land there are many scales to the turbulence. The largest scale would be induced by major obstacles such as hills and mountains, which would give rise to eddy interchanges up to thousands of feet, and would thus be responsible for bringing pathogenic particles (now freed of their raindrops) down to within hundreds of feet of the ground surface. Local irregularities, such as buildings and woodlands, generate intense fine-scale turbulence which can then reach upwards for these last remaining hundreds of feet. Local turbulent eddies generated by minor irregularities are therefore finally responsible for the detailed incidence of the pathogen at ground level. There may be fortunate spots which are either smooth enough or sheltered enough not to send local eddies upwards through these last remaining hundred feet or so. For these spots the pathogenic particles will fly by in the wind, immediately above the heads of people who fail to realise their good fortune.

Dr Briscoe told us that he is also the medical officer for St George's School, situated only a few hundred yards from Eton College. While Eton experienced an attack-rate of 35 per cent, St George's had no influenza at all. We think this was a case of St George's being located in one of the fortunate spots we have just mentioned. Fortunate spots may depend on wind direction, and so can shift around with the wind from one epidemic to another. Or a spot could be fortunate over a wide compass of the wind, like the school mentioned earlier that is high on a hill and rarely has epidemics. It is curious and not a little tragic that human societies tend to attach an imaginary morality to the incidence of disease, as if to say that a person catching a disease is somehow morally culpable, when indeed the issue may depend only on where we may happen to be situated in relation to local turbulence in the wind. For some places the pathogen simply blows safely by, for other places it strikes, as it struck at Latimer House, Headington (Table 6.3), and as it struck at Queenswood, Hatfield, whose Headmistress wrote to us: '... [I] can only say that in the first 48 hours (1st February–2nd February) 212 girls in the age range 11–18 were affected ...'

With these ideas in mind, we naturally took a look at meteorological data from mid-January to early March 1978, the period over which the epidemic attacks mainly occurred. Provided we avoided coastal regions, which were clearly affected by local squalls, the storm data at inland meteorological stations were generally similar from Cardiff in the west to Heathrow Airport, to Northampton, and up north into Yorkshire. We were therefore able to average the data for such inland stations without feeling that significant details were being lost. Unfortunately we had no local data for clearing skies, an essential part of our argument. Clearing skies are almost always associated with the passage of major fronts, however, and so we felt that if we constructed a numerical index suited to bringing out major frontal conditions we could expect to be also covering the requirement of clearing skies. The obvious daily index to choose was the product of the mean wind speed and of the precipitation. High values of the index would then imply both strong winds and heavy rain — i.e. frontal conditions. This we did for each day, and the results are shown in Figure 6.11. Then we constructed a histogram from the replies to our questionnaire showing the number of schools that reached the peak of the influenza attack on each day, and this histogram is given in Figure 6.12. The dates of the high peak of the meteorological index and of the schools histogram are set out in Table 6.5. The correspondence of dates, allowing for a three-day incubation period for the influenza, suggests, perhaps rather strongly, the existence of the kind of causal connection that we outlined above.

We end this chapter with a somewhat offbeat suggestion concerning the human nose. The human nose is not a directly

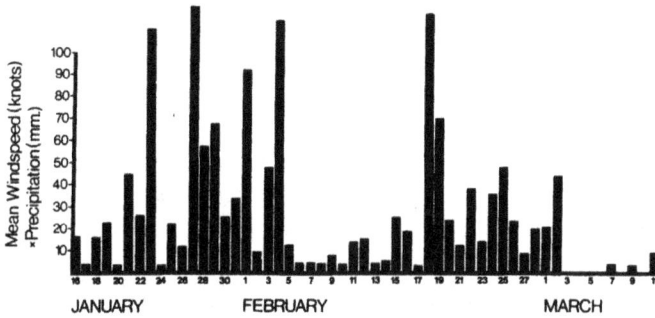

Fig. 6.11. Average of mean wind speed × precipitation data for several non-coastal meteorological stations.

Histogram of Peak Dates of Influenza Outbreaks

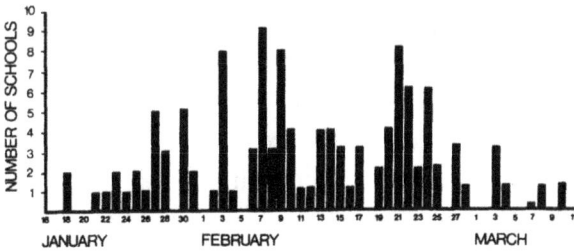

Fig. 6.12. Histogram of epidemic peak dates reported by schools in England and Wales.

Table 6.5. Dates of peaks of meteorological activity and of maxima of school influenza epidemics.

Meteorological activity	School influenza maxima
23 Jan	27 Jan
27 Jan	30 Jan
1 Feb	3 Feb
4 Feb	7–9 Feb
18–19 Feb	21–24 Feb

scaled-down version of an animal snout, such as is possessed by dogs, pigs, bears, cattle and so on — animals that have evolved out in the open. The human nose is a built-up version of an ape's nose, which consists externally of little beyond two adjacent holes in the face. An ape's nose is probably fine for a creature living in a forest, protected from infalling pathogens by a thick canopy of leaves overhead. But an ape's nose would be a poor thing for a creature that came out of the forest into open ground, since it would hardly be possible with such a nose to avoid the sniffing up of raindrops. Equipped only with two holes in the face, the incidence of pathogens could be an order of magnitude greater than it is with the human nose. An ape coming from the forest into the open therefore had to evolve a beak of a nose, from the end of which raindrops would drip rather than be sniffed up into the nasal passages.

It is very curious how much emotional importance we attach to the shape of the human nose, and how strongly significant it is in our assessment of a person's looks. This concern with nose shape could be a very old response, dating from times, hundreds of thousands of years ago, when the building of a substantial proboscis had become an important element in the fight against disease.

We began our thinking with the comparatively remote considerations of Chapter 2, with astronomical infra-red sources and with the acquisition of organic materials by the solar system as we discussed in our former book *Lifecloud*. Step by step we have progressed along a trail which has led us now to the shape of the human nose. A far more direct attack on the problem of disease could have begun with the nose itself. Pursued consistently, we think such an investigation would have led to just the same conclusion that we have reached, but in a reverse order. To produce a beak of a nose from two ape-like holes in the face, and to do so in a quite short time-scale of the order of a million years, demanded strong selection pressure. Selection pressure requires individuals that persisted genetically with ape-like holes in the face to die. Why should such individuals die? The human nose being a protection against breathing large liquid drops, we would need to infer that raindrops could on occasion be highly pathogenic. Why should this be? Because pathogens fall from the sky. So the argument would proceed, step by step backwards along the same trail that we have followed.

The evaluation of the human nose would also permit one to conclude that transmission from individual to individual has never been the dominant factor in the spread of disease, for transmission would have happened in the forest just as much as on open ground. It was therefore something which happened in open ground, something which could not be transmission, that generated heavy selection pressure for the human beak-nose. Moreover the population density throughout prehistoric times was low and could not have supported the reservoirs of bacteria and viruses that are required by the transmission hypothesis. Prehistoric populations were like small modern isolated communities, and it is one of the tenets of the transmission hypothesis that pools of disease die out in such communities — as on Tristan da Cunha.

Throughout the history of our species, open ground has been highly dangerous, unlike dense unbroken forest which afforded effective protection against the rain of pathogens from the sky. The rain of pathogens was not steady. It came in devastating bursts, the biggest bursts being separated by thousands of years. When the burst came, there was slaughter of animals on a vast scale, all over the open ground. Even animals with long snouts succumbed. In the first part of the next chapter we shall consider a remarkable quotation that will give us a valid impression of what happened on such occasions.

7

Isolation and Pandemics

A virus or bacterium incident on the Earth does not necessarily find itself a victim, and those that do will usually be restricted in their attack to a particular plant or animal. Yet there must be rarer cases where an attack spreads across two or more species. The influenza virus is particularly versatile in this respect, as will be seen from Table 4.2. As we expect, isolation of influenza virus from wild birds has been made frequently in recent years. Far-flying birds are especially subject to attack — they tend to find the patches of Figure 2.3.

Because no continuing reservoir of the influenza virus has been detected in humans, it has come to seem attractive to many epidemiologists to suppose that an influenza reservoir responsible for the human disease is carried by animals. For some years swine were thought to be the culprits, but the popular choice has swung nowadays from swine to birds. The jumping of the virus from bird to man, however, would need to be a rare event, otherwise the transfer process would be well-observed, which it has not been. Pandemics would therefore need to arise out of single transfer cases, thereby demanding an enormous multiplication of the disease by person-to-person transmission, a requirement that is contradicted by the evidence discussed in preceding chapters. In the second part of this chapter there will be references to epidemic attacks that occurred in ice-bound remote Alaskan villages during the late months of 1918. We leave the reader to wonder how birds could have caused these epidemics at such an advanced season of the year.

There are accounts in history showing that birds and other animals are themselves sometimes struck down by sudden attacks of influenza, just as decisively as humans are. In our view the infalling virus has no particular bias towards any one animal — it takes what it can get. Sometimes, as in 1918, the attack is devastating to man, and not so much to other animals. On other occasions the attack is devastating to an animal, as it was for poultry in 1927. The issue depends on the precise type of the virus. Wild birds are the biggest collectors of the virus, and being necessarily resistant to it, have the greatest number of subtypes temporarily resident within themselves.

A disease with symptoms resembling influenza is said to have attacked humans, dogs and birds in the year AD 876. Since the occurrence is reported in connection with the army of Charlemagne, it is likely to have been recorded by a responsible chronicler. Homer remarks on a similar incident at the beginning of the *Iliad:*

> Phoebus Apollo ... came down in fury from the heights of Olympus with his bow and covered quiver on his back. As he set out, the arrows clanged on the shoulder of the angry god; and his descent was like nightfall. He sat down opposite the ships and shot an arrow, with a dreadful twang from his silver bow. He attacked the mules first and the nimble dogs; then he aimed his sharp arrows at the men, and struck and struck again. Day and night innumerable fires consumed the dead.
>
> (*Trans.* E. V. Rieu)

It is of course a hazardous procedure to rely on the historical accuracy of the writings of a dramatic author. The plague which hits the Achaeans in the first pages of the *Iliad* has the eventual effect of dispatching Achilles in high dudgeon to his tent. This dispatching of Achilles is the pivotal device of the story, for without Achilles the Achaeans are just slightly inferior to the Trojans, whereas later, when Achilles at last joins the battle, the fine balance between the two sides is reversed, and the *Iliad* ends with the death and funeral rites of Hector, the Trojan leader. Homer's objective is to describe an epic struggle in which the only margin between the combatants resides in the fighting skills of just one man. In this way the poet keeps the struggle even, which is an essential condition, for if one side had clearly had the upper hand there would have been no worthwhile story. Seen in the context of the structure of the *Iliad,* the plague was clearly introduced by Homer as a stage-setting device, and so one must naturally be suspicious of its accuracy. Yet it is surely doubtful that any writer, however fictionally gifted, would have paused in a piece of stage-setting to invent the curious detail of the 'mules and nimble dogs'. They add nothing to the impressive quality of the moment. Indeed just the reverse, for there is more than a touch of the banal in the picture of the awesome Apollo loosing off his clanging arrows at mere mules and dogs. It seems more likely that Homer was drawing on a true situation which might well have been known to his audience, and which if it were so known would carry him smoothly through his piece of scene-setting.

Moving forward eight centuries, we come to a more extended quotation. Publius Vergilius Maro, Virgil to posterity, was a farmer's son. Born in 70 BC, he emerged around 38 BC as a poet of repute. In 37 BC, or thereabouts, he began the composition of a practical primer for the farmer, but written remarkably as a long and splendid poem. Towards the end of Book III of the *Georgics* he writes of the need for the shepherd to be constantly on the watch for the health of his flock:

> Now for the signs and causes of disease.
> Foul scab attacks the sheep when chilly rain
> And winter hoar-frost penetrate the flesh,
> Or unwashed sweat clings to the new-shorn flock,
> And prickly briars lacerate the skin.
> Wherefore the shepherds bathe them in the brook,
> And plunge the ram into the swirling pool,
> Letting his sodden fleece float down the stream,
> Or after shearing smear them with a salve
> Of bitter oil-lees, mixed with silver-scum

Pitch, natural sulphur, greasy wax and squill,
Black bitumen and stinking hellebore.
But there's no better remedy for this
Than boldly to incise the ulcer's head.
The mischief thrives so long as it is hid,
And, shrinking from the healing surgery,
The shepherd sits and prays for better luck.
Nay, when the sickness penetrates their bones,
And raging fever wastes away their flesh,
It's well to draw away the fiery heat
And lance a spurting vein within the hoof.
So the Bisaltae do and tough Gelonians,
That wander o'er the hills and wastes of Thrace,
And drink their milk curdled with horse's blood.
See you a sheep that seeks the kindly shade
And nibbles listlessly the tops of grass,
And lags behind and lies down in the field
While grazing, and returns home late at night?
Then check the evil with your knife at once,
Ere the contagion steal upon the rest.
The squalls that drive the storm in from the sea
Swoop not so thick and fast as pestilence,
That strikes not one by one but all the fold
At once, both sheep and lambs, and blasts your hopes.

How clearly speaks the farmer's son. Were the modern farmer suddenly stripped of his disinfectants and antibiotics he could do much worse than follow Virgil. So let us continue with the astonishing final passage of Book III of the *Georgics*. It is important to notice that the particular animals which Virgil mentions — dogs, birds, swine, horses, even cattle — are just the animals which modern research shows are attacked by the influenza virus (cf. Table 4.2). (It is also interesting that virus isolated from cattle in the Soviet Union has been found capable of infecting cattle elsewhere.) This correspondence of animal species suggests that the disease described by Virgil was indeed influenza, although there would also be bacterial secondary effects, and it suggests that his account of the disease was in all respects correct. At first sight, one might have suspicions about the four lines beginning. 'The vast deep's brood ...' Yet even here, it is relevant that there have been reports of antibody to Hong Kong virus found in seals, so that Virgil's reference to the 'seals that fled strangely up the river mouths' was probably well-founded. Also it is interesting to compare Virgil's 'shy deer and fleeting stags roamed round the houses ...' with the modern quotation from *The Lancet,* given at the end of Chapter 4, in which dead baboons were found in the vicinity of homesteads, 'the epidemic having caused them to forsake their usual haunts'. This is what Virgil says (Noricum is Austria):

Witness the wind-swept Alps and hill-top forts
Of Noricum and the Illyrian plains,
Where even now on every side you see
Abandoned pastures and deserted glades.

   'Twas here that once the tainted air brought forth
A plague that raged with all an autumn's heat.
It slew the herds and every kind of beast,
Infecting pools and poisoning pasture lands.
Death struck a double blow: first fiery thirst
Drove through their veins and shrivelled their poor limbs,
Then water humours spread, till all the bones
Were gradually rotted and absorbed.
Oft, as the victim at the altar stood
And round its head the snowy wool was tied,
It dropped down dead before the priest could strike.
Or, if the priest had struck the sacred blow,
The entrails would not burn upon the fire,
Nor could the soothsayer interpret them;
The knife beneath the throat was hardly wet,
The sand scarce darkened by the meagre gore.
The calves lay dying on abundant grass,
Or breathed their last beside full feeding troughs.
Good-natured dogs went mad; a breathless cough

Racked the sick swine and choked their swollen throats.
The once victorious horse, all spirit gone,
Forgetful of the pastures and the springs,
Continually stamped. His dropping ears
Broke into fitful sweat as cold as death;
His burning skin was dry and harsh to touch.
Such were the early signs of death's approach,
But, as the advancing sickness gathered strength,
Eyes grew inflamed and breathing deep and slow,
Broken by heavy sobs that shook his flanks.
His nostrils gushed with streams of dark-hued blood,
His tongue grew rough and blocked his swollen throat.
A draught of wine, poured through a drenching-horn,
Which often helps and seemed the only hope,
Soon led to death and only gave them strength
To rage with madness. For, though sick to death,
(Heaven grant good men a better remedy
And leave this error to our enemies!)
They rent their bodies with their own bare teeth.

    The smoking bull collapsed beneath the plough,
As blood poured from his mouth with mingled foam,
And heaved a dying groan. The ploughman sad
Unyoked the steer that mourned his brother's death,
And left the plough stuck in the half-worked field.
No deeply shaded grove, no meadow soft
Can touch his heart again, nor yet the stream,
That clear as amber skips among the stones.
His flank lies nerveless and his eye is glazed,
His neck sinks to the earth beneath its weight.
He toiled and served, and turned the heavy soil
To what avail? Yet he and such as he
Were never harmed by wine or revelry.
But leaves and simply grass are all their fare,
Their drink the limpid springs and hurrying streams,
Nor any care disturbs their healthy sleep.

    They say that in those parts, there never was
Before or since, a dearth of heifers fit

For Juno's rites, nor ill-matched buffaloes
Have drawn the chariots to her treasure-house.
Men scratched the soil with hoes and dug in seed
With their own nails, and dragged the creaking wains
Across the hills upon their straining necks.
The wolf tried not his wiles around the fold,
Nor prowled by night; an overpowering fear
Had made him tame. Shy deer and fleeting stags
Roamed round the houses and among the hounds.
The vast deep's brood and all the things that swim
Were cast like shipwrecked corpses on the shore,
And strangely seals fled up the river mouths.
Death found the viper in her hiding place,
The water-snake grew stiff with mortal fear.
The air was cruel even to the birds,
That falling headlong left their lives aloft.
Nor did it help to change the feeding-grounds,
And remedies wrought ill, nor aught availed
The skill of Chiron or Melampus' science.
From blackest hell pale-faced Tisiphone
Drove fear and Plague up to the light of day,
And ever higher reared her greedy head.
The thirsty river banks and sloping hills
Echoed with lowing kine and bleating sheep.
She dealt out death in droves, and in the stalls
Piled up the corpses, putrid with disease,
Until men learned to bury them in pits.
The hides could not be used, nor could the flesh
Be cleansed with water or subdued by fire.
They could not even shear or weave the wool,
So rotten that it crumbled at a touch;
And, if a man put on the loathsome garb,
Hot blisters broke out on his fetid limbs
And filthy sweat, and in a little while
The cursed fire was feeding on his joints.

We now come to our second major quotation. Read as a play
it has its hero in Thomas Riggs Jr, a man who maintains splendid

composure and coherence in the face of great provocation. Although Riggs, the Governor of Alaska, begins conventionally with the story that influenza was brought there 'following the line of steamship transportation', it is a very different picture that eventually emerges from his testimony, a picture of a huge territory over which the epidemic has spread, a territory much of it ice-bound, over which 'you only make 20 or 30 miles a day' by dog team. Boats did not bring the epidemic to Kodiak Island, since there were no boats to Kodiak.

This is a clear demonstration that birds are not responsible for spreading influenza. By November and December, the migratory flocks of Alaskan birds had long since moved far to the south, and the bird droppings of summer had long since been covered by the snows of winter.

When Riggs is cornered by several of the senators, over the sensitive point of the $600,000 in the Alaskan treasury, his protestations are highly relevant to our story. 'Our Indians ... have never been reservation Indians. They have been roving Indians ...' has critical importance in showing how influenza spread itself, not through a fixed static population, but through a thin nomadic population scattered over an intractable area 'two and a quarter times the size of the State of Texas'. Manifestly, this did not happen through a person-to-person transmission of the disease in conditions where you only made twenty of thirty miles in a day, and then only with the greatest difficulty: 'I have travelled over a great part of Alaska by dog team ...'

MONDAY, JANUARY 16, 1919
UNITED STATES SENATE,
COMMITTEE OF APPROPRIATIONS,
Washington, D.C.

The committee met at 2.30 o'clock p.m.
Present: Senators Martin (Chairman), Overman, Smith of Maryland, Smith of Arizona, Pollock, Smoot, Jones of Washington, Curtis, Kenyon and Calder.

Thomas Riggs, Jr, Governor of Alaska; Rupert Blue, Surgeon General of the Public Health Service; and Philander P. Claxton, Commissioner of Education, appeared.

The CHAIRMAN: The committee was called primarily to consider a joint resolution introduced by Senator Jones of Washington, appropriating $200,000 for the relief of the influenza sufferers in Alaska ...* Governor, we shall be glad to hear what you have to present about this matter.

Gov. RIGGS: Thank you, Senator. Perhaps I had better give you a brief history of how this happened.

Following the line of steamship transportation from Seattle, influenza broke out at first along the coast towns, and it rapidly extended to all of the small towns in south-eastern Alaska — all of the native villages, and the isolated communities. At Nome, which is in the northern part of Alaska, just before the freeze up — *when transportation ceased for the year* — influenza broke out; and, according to the last report I have, there have been approximately 1,000 deaths; 90 per cent of which were among the Eskimos. That has left on our hands over 150 Eskimo orphans. At the outlying places, like Kodiak, *where it was extremely hard to get assistance,* there were 40 or 50 deaths. There have been deaths *all over the Territory ...,* and the epidemic is still raging.

As to the Territorial funds, I had a fund of $5,000 only supplied by the Territory, which was expended almost before the epidemic started ... The expense of travelling in Alaska is enormous. I sent one doctor 400 miles by dog team to visit a stricken community. He got there, rendered what relief he could, and then was taken with the influenza himself and died, leaving all the lower Yukon River without any medical attention whatsoever ...

I felt it necessary to issue instructions to the officials of the Bureau of Education to do what they could for those who were starving, the destitute, the orphans, whether I had funds to do it with or not. I took the responsibility of that, hoping that Congress would grant me relief. The estimate of ... expenses incurred up to date is $107,000.

---

*We have taken the liberty of omitting parts of the report that were not relevant to our story, and we have set in italics the important remarks. Note that Senator Weeks is not listed among those present.

Sen. OVERMAN: Who represents the Surgeon General in Alaska?

Gov. RIGGS: The Surgeon General has several assistants. He has at present Dr Krolisch, of his office, who is doing what he can in looking after that part of Alaska *which is not frozen up.*

Sen. OVERMAN: *(Ignoring the unusual nature of the situation)*: It is unusual to allow the governor of a State or Territory to expend moneys in this regard when we have a department to expend the money. The work in this country has all been done by the Surgeon General, but I notice that this joint resolution asks that the money may be expended by the governor of Alaska.

Gov. RIGGS: Senator, I do not care by whom it is spent, so long as we get the relief. Somebody had to take the responsibility of doing it. The Surgeon General's office had not sufficient funds to enter into that work. It was a case of letting people starve and children perish unless I took that responsibility, and I took it. Whether I was wrong or not, I do not know; but I could not see people die.

Sen. SHAFROTH: Governor, have you heard as to the conditions up there at the present time?

Gov. RIGGS: I have a telegram here addressed to me under date of January 3 reading as follows:

'... Second epidemic about over on coast, excepting Cordova. Still raging along lower Yukon and Kuskokwim. Wire from Marshall today —

Marshall is on the lower Yukon River —

says 30 per cent native adult men died that vicinity. Unless funds supplied, purchase provisions, and maintenance, orphans, women, and children will starve. Dr Lamb died at Marshall.

He was the doctor I sent by dog team.

Have received no estimates quarantine expense interior towns or large coast towns. Shall I wire for their estimates? Mrs L. D. Henderson died last week.' She was the wife of the commissioner of education.

Sen. SHAFROTH: And she died of influenza?

Gov. RIGGS: She died of influenza; yes, sir.

Here is a telegram from Mr Evans, who is the assistant superintendent of the Bureau of Education at Nome.

'... Ten villages this district affected. Three wiped out entirely; others average 85 per cent deaths. Majority of children of affected villages saved by relief parties sent by the Bureau of Education. Teachers in stricken villages all sick; two dead; rest recovering. Total number of deaths reported 750; probably 25 per cent; this number frozen to death before help arrived. Over 300 children to be cared for, majority of whom are orphans ...

Appalling and beyond description ...

That is the condition at Nome.'

At Kodiak, which is an island in western Alaska, off towards the Aleutian Islands, they had some 300 cases of influenza; and owing to the fact that mail contracts had been cancelled there, there was no transportation.

Sen. SHAFROTH: How many died?

Gov. RIGGS: From the reports that I had about November 25, before leaving there, 40 had died and about 300 were ill. The naval collier *Brutus,* with officers of the Public Health Service, was sent up there, and afforded some relief. *That is the most northerly point that they can reach on account of ice conditions.* The rest of the Territory of Alaska has to be reached by dog team. The expense of travelling by dog team is terrific, and it is extremely difficult work. I know what travelling by dog team means. I have travelled over a great part of Alaska by dog team. *You have the short days, the hard, cold weather, and you only make 20 or 30 miles a day over the unbroken trails.* The conditions there are such as have never happened before in the history of the Territory.

Sen. SMITH of Arizona: How many people do you estimate live in Alaska now — I mean, the American population and the Indian population? Have you any means of knowing?

Gov. RIGGS: My estimate of the white population of Alaska this year is about 20,000 only. Two years ago it was about 45,000. They were drawn into the Army ...

Sen. SMITH of Arizona: *And if you keep up the 'conservation' that they have been practising up there, all the balance of them leave or die in the next few years.*

Sen. SMOOT: Governor, may I ask you a few questions about the estimated expense incurred? You stated that it was $107,000. Do I understand that that $107,000 is the estimate of expenses incurred under your order?

Gov. RIGGS: Under my order and the order of the Bureau of Education; yes, sir — the authorisations.

Sen. SMOOT: To what extent have the Bureau of Education ordered this expenditure of money?

Gov. RIGGS: They have asked me if I would authorise it, and just in the interest of humanity there I have taken the responsibility and said that I would authorise it.

Sen. SMOOT: The authorisation has always come from you?

Gov. RIGGS: From me; yes, sir.

Sen. SMOOT: Has the Territory paid anything towards this amount at all?

Gov. RIGGS: Only the $5,000 fund.

Sen. SMOOT: Have the people in Alaska assisted in any way?

Gov. RIGGS: The Red Cross chapters have spent all the money that they had on hand.

Sen. SMOOT: How much was that?

Gov. RIGGS: In the last Red Cross drive they raised approximately $160,000. Twenty-five per cent of that, or about $40,000, remained in the Territory.

Sen. SMOOT: What has the Government done?

Gov. RIGGS: Nothing, sir.

Sen. SMOOT: The Health Department of the Government has done nothing?

Gov. RIGGS: I beg your pardon; the Health Department of the Government has authorised the hiring of doctors and nurses where they could be obtained, and the purchase of medicines. I do not think the Health Department has had sufficient funds to authorise the carrying on of this (other) work.

Sen. KENYON: How much do you raise by territorial taxation?

Gov. RIGGS: We raise about half a million dollars.

Sen. SMITH of Arizona: What is the rate per cent of your taxation generally?

Gov. RIGGS: We have no rate per cent of taxation. Our taxes are raised principally on the production of salmon canneries — 4 cents per case of salmon. Then there are small taxes, which do not amount to much, on the net earnings of gold mines and on the net earnings of railroads and telephone companies; but, as I say, that does not amount to much. Our principal taxation is on fish. *(Continuing in the hope of getting the meeting back on course):* Gentlemen, you cannot conceive of what a terrible thing it is in that country, in wintertime, to have an epidemic, *with no means of getting around,* no doctors, no nurses, not even medical supplies, *because medicine cannot get there.*

The CHAIRMAN: What did you say the income from taxation in Alaska is, altogether?

Gov. RIGGS: The income from the Territorial taxation — I will give it to you exactly, Senator —

Sen. KENYON: You said half a million dollars.

Gov. RIGGS: I said *about* half a million dollars.

(*Determined now to be accurate*): The total receipts from all sources were $1,056,447.06. Total disbursements, various appropriations made by Territorial legislature, $373,953.95. Balance of cash on hand 31 December 1917, $682,493.11.

Sen. KENYON: What has become of all that surplus?

Gov. RIGGS: (*Resignedly letting the cat come out of the bag*): We have that balance on hand still in the Territorial treasury.

Sen. SMITH of Maryland: Over $600,000?

Gov. RIGGS: Over $600,000.

Sen. KENYON: Can you not have a special session of the legislature to take care of this matter?

Gov. RIGGS: It takes 45 days to call a special session of the legislature, and that would have been too late.

Sen. SMOOT: You have not any doubt, have you, that if you took the bull by the horns and spent $100,000 or $200,000 for this purpose, the legislature would back you up in it?

Gov. RIGGS: I really did not think so, Senator, but of course it is not a good thing to assume —

Sen. SMOOT: If they will not do that when they have the money in their own pockets, why should they come to the Government and ask the Government to do it?

The CHAIRMAN: You say there is about $600,000 in the treasury of Alaska now?

Gov. RIGGS: There is about $600,000 in the treasury of Alaska; yes, sir ... But there is this point: The United States Government does nothing for the Indians of Alaska. They are the only Indians in the United States who are not supported, if necessity arises, by the Government of the United States ...

The CHAIRMAN: (*Seeking to settle the matter without having his own committee involved*): You have the money there; the trouble is to get the legislature together to appropriate it? Is that the trouble? There is $600,000 in your treasury, so that you would not seem to be in any distress.

Gov. RIGGS: *(Stonewalling)*: Senator, it seems to be the opinion of the members of the Territorial legislature to whom I have talked that the Indians are not really the wards of the Territory; that the Indians are always considered the wards of the Government.

The CHAIRMAN: That is a rather strained idea. I do not see why the people there should not be taken care of, as far possible, by taxation.

Sen. SMITH of Arizona: I want to say, in justification of what the governor has said, that I have been through this for about 35 year, and when it comes to putting on 10,000 white people, with very little resources, the protection of forty, fifty, or sixty thousand Indians, they have no right to demand of the people of Alaska that any such thing shall be done. When the people of Alaska sustain the Alaskan government for themselves they have paid about all the taxes that any people on earth can bear.

The CHAIRMAN: ... We appropriated $215,000 (for Alaska last year).

Sen. SMITH of Arizona: For what?

The CHAIRMAN (Reading): To enable the Secretary of the Interior, in his discretion and under his direction, to provide for the education and support of the Eskimos, Aleuts, Indians, and other natives of Alaska; erection, repair, and rental of school buildings; text books and industrial apparatus; pay and necessary travelling expenses of superintendents, teachers, physicians, and other employees, and all other necessary miscellaneous expenses which are not included under the above special heads, $215,000.

Sen. SMITH of Arizona: That $215,000 is for the ordinary care of the Indians, as you state. With the Indians *scattered as they are in Alaska,* that is a very small item compared with what we give for the support and education of the Indians everywhere else — down in my country, and in Utah, and all through the West. It has been wrong from the start, and it is wrong now; but until we make a change closer home.

The CHAIRMAN: *(Not interested in a change nearer home)*: What difficulty is there in the way of using this $600,000 now in your treasury? Why cannot that be used for the relief of these people?

Gov. RIGGS: The people of Alaska consider that the money raised by taxes from the white people of Alaska should be spent for the improvements of the Territory. They need the money in roads a great deal. They want to spend more on roads; they want to spend more on the white schools; they want to spend more on their own sanitation;

... they want to have the Indians in Alaska placed more on a parity with the Indians of other parts of the United States where they are taken care of and looked after by the United States Government.

(In full voice): Our Indians are not given anything for their support. They get not 1 cent for support. They are self-supporting Indians. They have never been reservation Indians. *They have been roving Indians, and fishing and trapping Indians*, and have maintained themselves; and I would not be asking for any money for these Indians except for this epidemic that has swept *the whole Territory* and is causing all of this distress and devastation.

The CHAIRMAN: Referring to the $107,000 you have expended on this epidemic, what fund was that from?

Gov. RIGGS: There is no fund for it, Senator.

The CHAIRMAN: You must have gotten it from some fund. You said you have expended it.

Gov. RIGGS: I have *authorised* the expenditure. I have not spent it. I have authorised the expenditure. I have done that on my personal credit.

Sen. KENYON: Can you not keep on doing that until the legislature meets?

Gov. RIGGS: I can pay the bills I have already authorised. I am positive the legislature will not let me suffer any more than they have to; but then it is a question whether this should be properly charged against the Territory ...

Sen. KENYON: Governor, how much do you need, from now until the legislature meets, to take care of this particular influenza question?

Gov. RIGGS: I have a partial list which runs up to $107,500. I have 150 Eskimo orphans on my hands for whose support I have authorised the payment of $10 a month each. I have perhaps a thousand Indians unburied, and the best price I can get — they have to thaw the ground for graves with steam — is $30 an Indian.

Sen. KENYON: Governor, you did not answer my question. How much money do you need now to carry this work on until the legislature meets approximately?

Sen. SMOOT: You have January and February — two months.

Sen. KENYON: Yes. Now, how much do you need to get through this time? I do not care for what you have authorised. Cut that out.

Gov. RIGGS: I will need $150,000 ...

Sen. KENYON: You have not any doctors there, have you?

Gov. RIGGS: We have very few doctors. We have an Indian doctor at a place called Nulaka, on the Yukon River, and then for 500 miles either way we have not a doctor.

Sen. KENYON: *(Forgetting the cost of burials, the orphans, and the destitute)*: Just what do you do with the money? You have no doctors; you have no nurses.

Sen. WEEKS: *(In deep tones)*: Mr Chairman, do you contemplate passing that appropriation of $100,000,000 to feed the people of Europe?

The CHAIRMAN: I shall support it myself. I do not know what the Congress will do with it.

Sen. WEEKS: *(Instantly putting a stop to it all)*: I think we might take whatever appropriation is required for this purpose out of that.

The CHAIRMAN: Do you think this is as important as that?

Sen. SHAFROTH: If we are going to feed foreigners it seems to me we ought to feed our own people.

Sen. JONES: I think so, too.

Sen. SMOOT: *(With a last attempt to nit-pick)*: It is not a question of feeding them; it is a question of taking care of them.

Sen. SHAFROTH: *(With welcome good sense)*: It is a question of preserving their lives or letting them starve to death.

Sen. JONES: It is a good deal a matter of feeding them, too.

Gov. RIGGS: *(Seeing that he had won)*: There is a good deal of feeding to be done, too, Senator.

Sen. SMOOT: *(Seeing that he has lost)*: Do you want to say anything more?

The CHAIRMAN: Is there anything else, Governor?

Gov. RIGGS: No; except that I sincerely hope this committee will grant the relief that I am asking, because the epidemic is not over; it is spreading. *It is spreading to regions that we thought we had barred off but they are not barred off,* and the epidemic is not half over.

(As a Parthian Shot): I should like to draw your attention, if I may, for just one minute, to the action of the Canadian Government. When they heard that there was influenza in Alaska and on the coast, without waiting for the influenza to reach their own natives, they sent out patrols of the Northwest Mounted Police loaded with medical supplies, and they were told not to come home until they had controlled the epidemic and it was over, without any limit as to how far they should go.

8

Plagues Past and Present

Human diseases caused by bacteria and viruses must be as old as man himself. We have already pointed out that microbial invasions from space started about 3.5 billion years ago with the injection of cometary material on to the Earth. This process, which initially led to the origin of life on our planet, must have continued unabated ever since. With the evolution of plants and animals of ever-increasing complexity, some of these later microbial invasions must have been pathogenic. It is likely that microbes which had the potential of causing human disease began to arrive here well ahead of our emergence as a species. In our view, man must have evolved so as to adapt continually to invading microbes, even at times assimilating some into his genetic heritage. This scheme seems more likely to us than the usual view of microbes adapting to man.

What record do we have of early human diseases, either viral or bacterial? And is there evidence for a changing pattern of disease, as we would indeed expect on the basis of our hypothesis? In the present chapter we shall attempt to find answers to some of these questions from a historical record which must of necessity be somewhat fragmentary and incomplete.

In previous chapters we have discussed at some length the behaviour of two viral diseases, the common cold and influenza. We found evidence to support the view that the causative viruses for each of these diseases come directly from space, settling through the atmosphere in a patchy distribution. Every new epidemic of such diseases would appear to be driven from outside. A pristine virus, one that originates in a comet, must be encased in a protective matrix which could be an inorganic grain, an organic particle or even a bacterium, in order for it to survive the journey to Earth. The ingestion of such a virus particle by a human host then leads in some cases to the stripping of the matrix and to subsequent replication and multiplication of a naked virus. The influenza or common cold virus which is thus released from an infected person has a very short lifetime. Exposed to sunlight and air a naked influenza virus becomes inactivated in a matter of hours. No long-term reservoir of virus can be established, nor is there any possibility of appreciable transfer of virus from person to person.

Other diseases for which the causative viruses also have a cometary origin could behave differently. Pathogenic viruses isolated in some diseases are found to be more robust and more persistent than others. Whereas the free influenza virus is viable only for a matter of hours under normal conditions, the virus which causes smallpox may have a lifetime that is measured in tens of years. The more robust viral species could establish long-term reservoirs in a host population more easily. For diseases in which a single attack confers lifelong immunity to a surviving host, the maintenance of an infective reservoir requires the fulfilment of two conditions. New births must occur at a fast enough rate to provide a replacement of susceptible persons, and large enough concentrations of susceptibles who are in communication with one another must be maintained. Such concentrations of population would not have occurred in palaeolithic societies where man lived basically as a hunter and food gatherer, constantly on the move and widely scattered over the globe in small groups. Most of the infective diseases affecting such groups were probably due to the incidence of pristine viruses, with no possibility of either transmission or storage for a long time

Modern man is besieged by a great variety of microbial species that can cause disease. Some of these microbes may be truly pristine — in other words they may come from space *de novo*. Others may have come initially from space at some time in the past, but now they have established reservoirs from which fresh infections can spring forth, with the disease then being passed from person to person (or animal to person) during epidemics. There could also be an intermediate category of disease where a long-term microbial reservoir is established and where such a reservoir is periodically replenished or 'topped up' from outside. To which of these three categories do familiar diseases belong? Does a given type of disease microbe have:

(1) no terrestrial reservoir,
(2) a reservoir established at some time in the past with no subsequent replacement, or
(3) a reservoir which is periodically 'topped up' from outside?

Starting from the known symptoms and effects of some present-day diseases we shall now follow the history of these diseases in an attempt to trace their origins as well as to determine the categories to which they belong.

Diseases which can be traced furthest back in time are those which leave distinctive marks on the human skeleton. The virus-caused disease poliomyelitis is an example. The acute phase of this disease involves muscular paralysis. But skeletal deformities such as shortening of a limb or a club foot are frequently a late result, particularly in cases where the disease is contracted in childhood. A shortened femur, characteristic of poliomyelitis, was found in a skeleton of an Egyptian pre-dynastic mummy which was dated by J. K. Mitchell in 1900 as over 5000 years old. There are also much later artistic depictions of shortened limbs surviving from the Eighteenth Dynasty in Egypt. A considerable body of circumstantial evidence thus points to the presence of poliomyelitis as a human disease at least as far back as 3000 BC. This disease is also described by Hippocrates in his discussion of epidemics.

Epidemic outbreaks of polio, affecting young children in the main, continued to occur periodically throughout the world until 1961, when an effective vaccine was prepared. In 1955 there were 31,582 cases of paralytic polio recorded in the United States. Since the introduction of a live polio virus vaccine followed by the Salk vaccine, this number has rapidly dwindled. During the three-year period 1973–1975 only 20 cases of paralytic poliomyelitis occurred in the United States. A similar pattern has emerged in most developed countries where vaccination programmes have

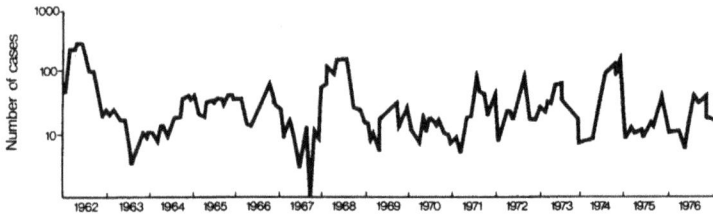

Fig. 8.1. Incidence of Poliomyelitis in Sri Lanka (data supplied by Dr P. U. de la Motte, Epidemiologist, Ministry of Health, Colombo).

been implemented and maintained. Although paralytic polio is practically non-existent in these countries, it still continues to affect many developing countries where the implementation of vaccination programmes is still incomplete. Figure 8.1 shows the incidence of paralytic polio in Sri Lanka during the period 1962–1976. A rather precise six-year periodicity which shows up here has also been noted in the Indian state of Kerala. Since there is no significant movement of people between Kerala and Sri Lanka, there is evidence here of a periodic 'topping up' of a viral reservoir over a fairly large geographical area. We would thus predict that if polio immunisation were stopped in the more advanced countries, a poliomyelitis viral reservoir would be quickly re-established and the old disease patterns would reappear.

The discovery of pockets of polio in totally isolated population groups also suggests a continuing external input of virus. The Trio are a group of Amerindians living in dense forests near the equator in northern Brazil and southern Surinam. This terrain, which is amongst the harshest in the tropics, has for long been preserved from exploration because of the impenetrable thickness of surrounding forest as well as rapid unnavigable rivers. Furthermore, the tribes inhabiting these regions are bow-hunters with a reputation for atrocities which had daunted many a prospective explorer. Forest clearings initiated by the Surinam government began in the late 1950s and by the early 1960s the Trio came under the scrutiny of the outside world. To the surprise of the medical profession it was found that poliomyelitis was present in these regions. Several cases of polio-induced paralysis were found in persons whose ages and histories placed the incidence of the disease to a date well before the clearing of the forest. There could have been no conceivable chance that the Trio tribe were infected by people outside their forest dwelling.

The bacillus-caused disease tuberculosis is another disease which leaves its imprint on the skeletons of victims. The disease in its chronic form is not confined to the lungs and often causes bony lesions. Dr Morse and his colleagues have found such evidence which points to tuberculosis in ancient Egypt as far back as 3700 BC. Experts, however, are not convinced by these data because other diseases could also cause rather similar bony lesions. Unequivocal evidence of tuberculosis has been found in the lungs of an Egyptian mummy of the Twenty-first Dynasty dated at about 1000 BC. The disease was also most probably known in India at around 1300 BC. The *Ordinances of Manu* compiled at about this time carry an admonition to bridegrooms to be cautious of marrying into a family which is prone to the disease. An unambiguous description of tuberculosis is given in *Sushruta Samhita,* an Indian compilation dated at around the sixth century BC. The disease was also known to Hippocrates and to other Greek and Roman medical commentators after the fifth century BC. Tuberculosis is evidently a very old disease, one for which a pathogenic reservoir has been stably held in a human population for several thousand years.

Few human diseases can be more disfiguring and crippling than leprosy. Like tuberculosis this is also a bacillus-caused disease. Victims of leprosy have had to endure the most ruthless social ostracism in addition to suffering the gruesome horrors of the disease itself. The Old Testament contains several clear descriptions of leprosy which date a presence of the disease at about 1300 BC. Leprosy is also clearly recognisable in the *Charaka Samhita,* the Indian medical treatise written in about 600 BC. Yet somewhat surprisingly there is no reference to leprosy in the Hippocratic writings and in later Greek and Roman medical writings until the second century AD. A possible explanation of this lack of reference is that the disease disappeared at around the fifth century BC and that it reappeared in Europe early in the Christian era. Leprosy seems to have been clearly described by Galen in the second century AD, and there is evidence of its ravages on an Egyptian mummy of the sixth century AD.

The viral disease trachoma, which causes great suffering and often leads to total blindness, is still present in many tropical and subtropical countries, as well as in certain parts of the United States. The infection causes eyes to burn and ooze constantly and vision blurs. The eyelids become crusty and distorted and corneas develop scars which lead to blindness. The disease is first described in the Papyrus Ebers which was written 1500 years before Christ. It is said to have plagued Egypt for several centuries some 3500–4000 years ago. A description of trachoma is also to be found in the Hippocratic writings, but the disease was then probably much less prevalent than it was in ancient Egypt. If one takes the historical evidence at face value, we have in trachoma a disease which assumed severe pandemic proportions 4000 years ago, but which has since steadily diminished in incidence despite the increasing concentrations of people in cities. A viral reservoir which was continually being resupplied from space over a 500-year period in ancient Egypt would appear to have slowly decayed during the subsequent period of nearly three millennia.

There is considerable uncertainty on the origins and antiquity of the bacillus-caused disease cholera. It seems most likely that the disease was non-existent before AD 1519, but this statement must be regarded as tentative. More definitely we can say that cholera has a characteristic set of symptoms which are nowhere on record before this date. Cholera causes violent fits of vomiting, diarrhoea, painful muscle cramps, unquenchable thirst, feeble pulse and blood pressure and very low body temperature. The mortality is high, varying between 15 per cent and 75 per cent, the higher rate being valid for epidemics. Today the disease is endemic to two major foci, the delta of the River Ganges in India and the El Tor district of Sinai. Conditions prevalent in these regions — humid heat, a low-lying terrain with a high water table, and dense concentrations of people — appear favourable for maintaining a stable reservoir for the cholera-causing bacillus. Nevertheless, the disease is not always confined to endemic foci. Sporadically, and often quite mysteriously, epidemic outbreaks of cholera occur well outside the confines of these main foci.

Pandemics of cholera have sporadically swept across Asia, Africa, the Middle East, Europe and America, claiming millions of lives. Such pandemic outbreaks usually lasted for thirty to fifty years and then retreated as swiftly and as mysteriously as they came. A cholera pandemic of a particularly lethal type began in India in 1817. Victims were reported to have died within a day of being attacked. Between 1817 and 1850 cholera had spread across almost the entire world. The death-rate topped 15 per cent in several affected areas, and many millions of people are believed to have died. In 1851 the pandemic appeared to retreat, but there were several subsequent returns. The later invasions were somewhat less devastating mainly because the causative bacillus had been isolated and the mode of spread of the disease had been discovered. The Frenchman Felix Pouchet isolated *vibries,* the bacillus causing cholera, from the stool of a patient in 1849, and at about the same time the Englishman John Snow discovered that the bacillus was water borne. Snow had noticed that within a 250 yard radius of a public water pump at the intersection of Broad and Cambridge Streets in London, some 500 people had died of cholera within a period of ten days. Many of the victims were people who drank regularly at this water pump, often using the water to mix drinks obtained at nearby pubs. There was thus a strong suggestion of a causal connection between cholera and the water supply. As Snow writes in *On the Mode of Communication of Cholera,* published in 1849:

> ... When the water of a river becomes infected with the cholera evacuations emptied from on board ship, or passing down drains and sewers, the communication of the disease ... is much more widely extended ... I know of no instance in which it has been generally spread through a town or neighbourhood, among all classes of the community, in which drinking water has not been the medium of its diffusion ...

With the removal of the water pump at Broad Street the epidemic stopped and Snow's suspicions were confirmed.

Epidemics of cholera have continued to occur at irregular intervals in various parts of the world. From among the unidentified throng of sufferers, the ciphers of history, a face stands out clear and sharp — the Russian musician Tchaikovsky. Today, however, cholera is not a life-threatening disease when it is competently handled. Medical treatment involves careful rehydration of the patient combined with the administration of antibiotics. Precautions and preventive measures against contracting the disease are also sufficiently easy to take. For example, the precaution of drinking boiled water combined with simple rules of hygiene are adequate in places where the disease is endemic, or during epidemics. Vaccinations made from heat-killed bacterial cultures afford some measure of immunity, but resistance to the disease is usually short-lived, lasting for no more than six months.

The periodic surges of cholera occurring in pandemic proportions are difficult to understand in terms of the orthodox theory of infectious diseases. Just at the time when cholera was thought to be on the verge of extinction a pandemic broke out in 1961, affecting twenty countries in Asia, the Middle East and the Far East. In our view such global onslaughts of cholera as occurred in the nineteenth century as well as later must represent fresh invasions from outside, in which transient reservoirs of the cholera bacillus become established outside the confines of the two endemic foci.

Measles, a childhood disease which is caused by a virus, presents many interesting problems. It is considered to be highly infectious, with an incubation period of about fourteen days. A single attack confers lifelong immunity, and man is the only known host for this virus. A continuing prevalence of the disease in any community depends therefore on the steady supply of new susceptibles from births or migrations, the density of such susceptibles being maintained at a sufficiently high value to permit person-to-person transmission. Alternatively, or in conjunction with the transmission process, fresh supplies of the virus could be introduced periodically from outside.

The symptoms of measles, including its characteristic rash, are not likely to go unrecognised if the disease existed at any time in the past. The fact that there is no description of measles either in Hippocrates (fifth century BC) or in the Indian medical writings of the sixth century BC may be interpreted as implying the absence of the disease during this period. Epidemics of measles may possibly have occurred in the Roman Empire in AD 165 and in China in AD 162. The Persian doctor Abu El Rhazes, who lived AD 860–932, has provided the first clear description of the disease. From Rhazes's reference to earlier literature, it is clear that measles already existed at least 300 years before his time. It is interesting that Rhazes considered measles to be a serious illness 'more to be dreaded than smallpox, except in the eye'. Rhazes also observed the seasonal nature of measles, but he did not consider the disease to be infectious.

Person-to-person infection through coughing and sneezing of viral particles is considered to be the most likely way in which measles is propagated during epidemics, but there is no firm evidence to support this view. The disease occurs in temperate countries with a distinct seasonality. The first cases of measles begin to appear in late February or early March and the epidemic usually reaches a peak in March–April. Evidence of a March peak in the annual incidence of this disease in London can be traced back to AD 1670. Spring epidemics are usually attributed to the start of school sessions, but such an association is most likely to be coincidental. There is no evidence of similar epidemics in the winter or summer terms. A typical annual incidence curve of measles is shown in Figure 8.2. In addition to the annual March–April peaks, there are oscillations in the intensity of annual epidemics with periods in the range 3–5 years.

These facts about measles are usually fitted into orthodox epidemiological theory in a rather contrived way. The annual occurrence of March epidemics is attributed to a seasonal variation in the viability of the measles virus. A virus particle coughed out in March is postulated to survive for significantly longer than one exuded at any other time of the year. And the 3–5 years periodicities

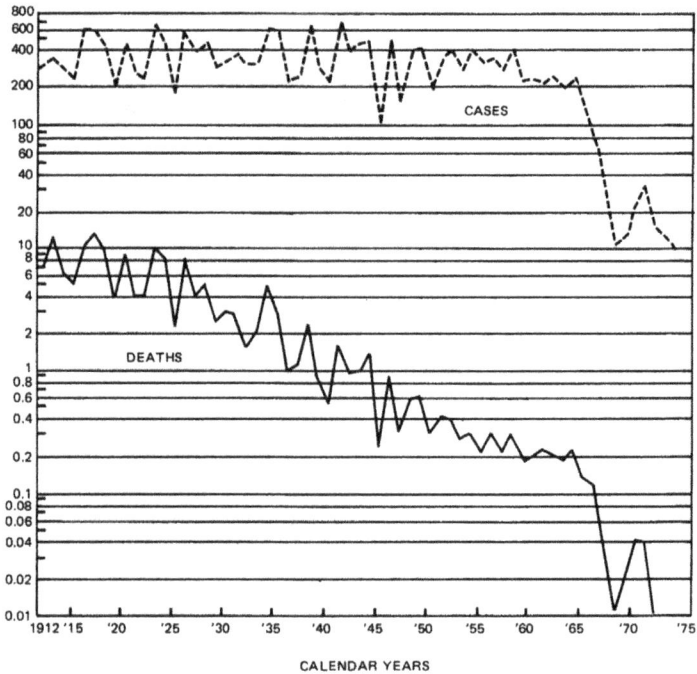

Fig. 8.2. Incidence curve for measles (from *Viral Infections of Humans,* ed. A. S. Evans, Wiley, 1976).

are identified with the time required for newly born children to regenerate a high density of susceptibles to the disease. In our view the measles virus is likely to have a direct space origin with no need for a long-term terrestrial reservoir. An annual incidence could be associated with meteorological events which bring the virus down from the stratosphere. The 3–5 years periodicity could be the time lag associated with the build-up of a new population of susceptibles, or it could be associated with a periodic incidence of cometary particles. The first entry of measles virus to the Earth seems to have occurred around AD 160, and during the first few hundred years the disease appears to have been exceptionally virulent.

Another childhood disease, mumps, is also caused by a virus and is clearly described in the Hippocratic writings:

Although the climate was generally southerly and dry, in the early spring there was a northerly spell, the very opposite of the previous weather. During this time a few people contracted *causus* without being much upset by it, and a few had haemorrhages but did not die of them. Many people suffered from swellings near the ears, in some cases on one side only, in others both sides were involved. Usually there was no fever and the patient was not confined to bed. In a few cases there was slight fever. In all cases the swellings subsided without harm and none suppurated as do swellings caused by other disorders. The swellings were soft, large and spread widely, they were unaccompanied by inflammation or pain and they disappeared leaving no trace. Boys, young men and male adults in the prime of life were chiefly affected ...

Whether it existed before the fifth century BC and for how long is not known. It seems likely that the causative virus for mumps has established a terrestrial reservoir which is periodically replenished from outside.

The beginnings of chickenpox or varicella are difficult to trace. This is mainly because of the difficulty of differentiating between a mild attack of smallpox and chickenpox without recourse to virological investigations. Two viruses, however, *herpes simplex* and *herpes zoster,* which are either very closely related to or identical with chickenpox, are of considerable antiquity. The virus *herpes simplex* causes eruptions on the lips and nose which are called 'cold sores'. Eruptions of cold sores were described by the Roman physician Herodotus at around AD 100. Another Roman physician, Scribonius Largus, writing at about the same time, refers to symptoms characteristic of shingles, a disease caused by the virus *herpes zoster.* The description of an eruption of vesicles in the form of a narrow band around the trunk makes this disease clearly recognisable. Since we know now that an attack of shingles can be triggered by exposure to chickenpox, we can infer that chickenpox was also probably present around the first century AD.

The Herpes group of viruses are of particular interest because of their exceptionally long-term persistence in a host. People who have been once infected can carry the virus in a latent yet viable form throughout their lives. The implication is that a reservoir once supplied from outside could be maintained in a population for tens of thousands of years or even longer. Herpes viruses may therefore be amongst the oldest microbial invaders of our planet.

Bubonic plague caused by the bacterium *Pasteurella pestis* is another quite ancient and mysterious human affliction. This bacillus parasitises on many species of rodent, but most epidemics of human plague have been caught from the black rat which tends to infest human habitations. The disease is thought to be conveyed to humans by fleas which bite an infected rat and then a human victim. The earliest, albeit rather ambiguous, reference to plague appears in the Old Testament. The Philistines were said to have been attacked by a plague involving 'emrods [plague buboes] in their secret parts ...' as a reprisal for stealing the Ark of God belonging to the Hebrews. If this is indeed a factual reference to an outbreak of the bubonic plague, the likely date is about 1200BC. The first definite reference to plague occurs in the *Bhagavata Purana,* an Indian medical treatise written in the fifth century. There is a clear warning for people to leave their houses 'when rats fall from the roofs above, jump about and die'. Rufus of Ephesus gives a description of what was most likely an outbreak of plague in Syria and North Africa during the first century AD.

Between the first and sixth centuries AD there were no known outbreaks of bubonic plague, the next outbreak occurring in AD 540 during the reign of the Roman Emperor Justinian. A major pandemic of plague spread throughout the Near East, North Africa and southern Europe, causing deaths on a scale hitherto unseen. The English historian Edward Gibbon thought it likely that the death toll reached 100 million. Between 5000 and 10,000 people are thought to have died daily at Constantinople alone. The contemporary historian Procopius described the plague thus:

> They were taken with a sudden fever: some suddenly wakened from sleep; others while they were occupied with various matters during daytime. The fever, from morning to night, was so slight that neither the patient nor the physician feared danger, and no one

believed that he would die. But in many even on the first day ...
a bubo appeared both in the inguinal regions and under the
armpits ... Some died at once, others after many days, and the
bodies of some broke out with black blisters the size of a lentil.
These did not live after one day, but died at once, and many were
quickly killed by a vomiting of blood ... Physicians could not tell
which cases were light and which severe, and no remedies availed.

The Plague of Justinian lasted about fifty years.

For the next 800 years the world seems to have been mercifully
spared from the ravages of plague. If *Pastuerella pestis* continued
to parasitise on rodents there must have been stringent controls
on the rodent and/or flea populations which were maintained with
an uncanny precision throughout eight centuries. A much more
plausible explanation is that the bacterial reservoir disappeared, the
bacterium *Pasteurella pestis* being an irregular visitor to our planet.

The next pandemic of the plague came in the form of the 'Black
Death' in the fourteenth century. The massacre which ensued was
on a scale that the world had never before seen. Countless millions
died. Much of the world was literally strewn with corpses, a scene
which persisted for nearly three centuries. The Plague of London of
1664 is believed to have been one of the final epidemic outbreaks
of this long drawn-out pandemic. Then followed another plague-
free period which lasted for about 230 years. The most recent phase
of the bubonic plague started in China in 1894. Between 1896 and
1917 it spread into India, killing some 13 million people.

Figure 8.3 is a map due to Dr E. Carpentier, showing the
spread of the Black Death across Europe. Compiled from historical
records of the first outbreaks of the disease in various centres of
population, the map shows that there is a great deal wrong with
the usual explanations of how the Black Death moved from place
to place.

Since the contours give the dates of the *first* outbreak of the
Black Death at the various locations, it is impossible that two
different ones should intersect. Yet this is the situation towards
which the contours for December 1347 and December 1348 appear

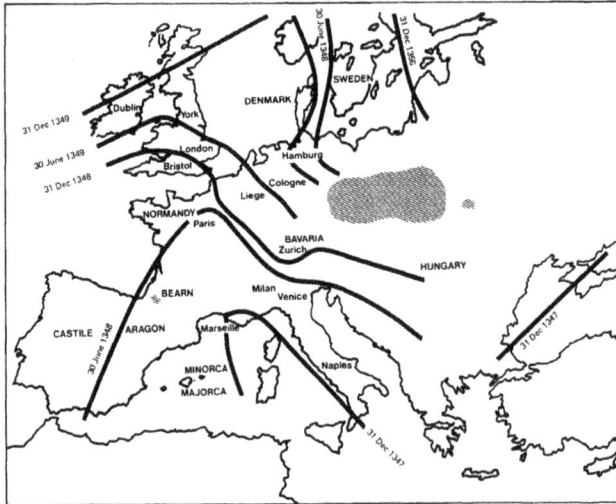

Fig. 8.3. The spread of the Black Death through Europe (after Dr E. Carpentier).

to be heading (in the region of the Danube delta). The suspect contour is the earlier one, which seems to have been drawn, not from reliable documentary evidence as with the later contours, but in order to conform with the story that *Pastuerella pestis* reached Europe from Asia.

The tale is that the Tartars, while besieging a Genoese base at Caffa in the Crimea, catapulted the corpses of plague victims in amongst the defenders, who thereupon contracted the disease which they then brought with little delay by ship to western Italy. The December 1347 line marks the voyage of the Genoese. This story must be wrong, however, because the plague was not transmitted by corpses, a fact that was eventually made plain in every European city, where those who collected the dead from the houses did not turn out to be more susceptible to the disease than anybody else. The reason we know today is that the fleas which carry *Pasteurella pestis* from rats to man quit the bodies of dead victims. The catapultor rather than the Genoese would have got the fleas.

The successive half-yearly contours of Figure 8.3 are interpreted by orthodox opinion as steps in the march of an army of plague-infected rats. Humans with the disease collapsed on the spot, and we think afflicted rats must surely have done the same. To argue that stricken rats set out on a safari that took them in six months not merely from southern to northern France, but even across the Alpine massif, borders on the ridiculous. Nor does the evidence by any means support in detail such an inexorable stepwise advance of the plague. Pedro Carbonell was the archivist to the Court of Aragon, a pose that in its very nature could only be held by a person with a clear appreciation of the difference between fact and fiction. Carbonell reports that the Black Death began in Aragon, not at the Mediterranean coast or at the eastern frontier, but in the western island city of Teruel.

Since it apparently stretches credulity too far to argue that the advancing army of stricken rats also managed to swim the English Channel, it is said that the Black Death reached England by ship. Yet the contours of Figure 8.3 are of quite the wrong shape for boats to have played a significant role in spreading the disease. If *Pasteurella pestis* had been carried by sea, the contours would have had the shape of Figure 8.4, with the earliest one spread around the coast, and with subsequent contours filling in gradually towards central Europe. Not only this, but if the bacillus had travelled by sea, the coast of Portugal would have been seriously affected. One historian remarks: 'Until recently it was the tradition that the plague scarcely penetrated to Castile, Galicia and Portugal. *This is clearly not true ...*' Why it is 'clearly not true' our historian does not trouble to explain. His concern of course is to fit the advancing rat theory, not to fit the evidence. But to say so explicitly would have been embarrassing to his own profession.

There are many descriptions of communities that isolated themselves deliberately from the outside world, and many of these descriptions come from English villages. Yet isolation was to no avail. The Black Death would strike suddenly, and within a week the people in such communities would be in just the same dire straits as everyone else. Recent amendments to the old records almost always

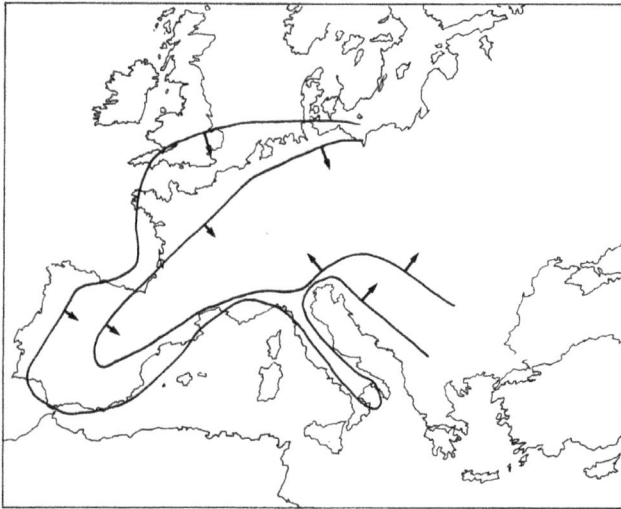

Fig. 8.4. If the Black Death had been spread by sea, the outer line would have been earlier than the inner line, with the disease spreading in the directions of the arrows.

seek to tell us of a solitary intruder from the outside world who, it is said, managed somehow to slip past the community guard, so bringing in the disease. The inventors of these embroideries show their inexperience by mistakenly casting the intruder as a human instead of as a rat.

What remarkable rats they were. To have crossed the sea and to have reached into remote English villages, and yet to have effectively by-passed the cities of Milan, Liège and Nuremberg! To have largely spared an extended area in Bohemia and southern Poland, as well as smaller pockets in western Europe. The astonishing reason offered for this behaviour is indicative of the state of mind engendered by orthodox theory. The rats, it is said, disliked the food available to them in these regions.

We remarked above that Indian doctors had noticed already in the fifth century the connection of plague with rats. Yet medieval doctors had no such thoughts. It was their overwhelming view that the pestilence had its origin in the air — 'poisoned' air was the widely favoured explanation. It has been fashionable to decry this view as an unsubstantiated superstition, although the state of technical understanding in fourteenth-century Europe was higher than it had been at any earlier stage of human history. Modern commentators have ignored the ideas of medieval doctors on the ground that medical and scientific knowledge was then primitive. Yet this may have been the very circumstance that permitted doctors to stumble unwittingly upon a profound truth. There was no overpowering edifice of scientific theory to stifle imagination, nor was there a scientific orthodoxy that influenced a sifting of those correlations which were respectable from those which were not.

If one is not irredeemably prejudiced by modern superstitions, the contours of Figure 8.3 are a clear indication that *Pasteurella pestis* hit Europe from the air. There was no marching army of plague-stricken rats. The rats died in the places where they were infected, just as humans did. By falling from the air, *Pastuerella pestis* had no difficulty at all in crossing the Alps, or in crossing the English Channel. Remote English villages were hit, however determinedly they sought to seal themselves off from the outside world, because the plague bacillus descended upon them from above; and against an aerial assault all the precautions taken were of no consequence. Milan, Liège and Nuremberg were comparatively unscathed because it is in the nature of incidence from the upper atmosphere that there will be odd spots where a pathogen does not fall, as in the picture of Figure 2.3. So too did Bohemia and southern Poland escape, even though these areas grew food just as palatable (we think) to rats as everywhere else.

As in the case of bubonic plague, the causative micro-organism for smallpox is almost certainly a recurrent visitor to our planet. Smallpox, being highly infectious, is one of the most dreaded of human diseases for which there is neither cure nor treatment. On the average, four in ten smallpox victims die of the disease, and survivors are covered with disfiguring pock marks. Man is the only known host for the smallpox virus, which has such an exceptionally long persistence that corpses of smallpox victims remain infectious for many years. There are well-documented records of people being infected from such corpses after thirty years of burial (P. Razell, 1977).

The ultimate origins of smallpox are lost in the mists of antiquity. Lesions in the skins of Egyptian mummies of the eleventh century BC bear a striking resemblance to smallpox. Vedic literature of India, dated at about the same time, also refers to inoculation procedures which were most probably against smallpox: '... put liquid from the pustulis on to the point of a needle, and introduce it into the arm, mixing the liquid with the blood. A fever will be produced, but this illness will be mild, and should cause no alarm ...' There is also some fairly slender evidence which suggests that smallpox was present in China at the same time. The Jesuit missionary Cibot stated that at the Imperial Palace in Peking, he had seen a book entitled *Treatise from the Heart on Smallpox,* in which reference was made to the disease first appearing at the time of the Tsche-U Dynasty, 1122–249 BC (Moore, 1815). If smallpox was indeed present in the eleventh century BC, as the evidence strongly suggests, it is equally clear that it was not present in either India or Europe in the fifth and sixth centuries BC.

There is no reference to smallpox in either the Hippocratic writings or in the Indian medical treatises, *Charaka Samhita* and *Sushruta Samhita,* completed around 600 BC. Smallpox seems to have made its next appearance very early in the Christian era after skipping a millennium. It was almost certainly prevalent in China in AD 49 (Smith, 1871), and the so-called Antonine pestilence which raged through the Roman Empire in the second century AD is recognisable as smallpox from the description given by Galen. Again, mysteriously, it disappears for some 400 years. In view of the severity of the disease and its strongly disfiguring property, an absence of reference by writers in the early Christian era almost certainly implies absence of the disease.

The next appearance of smallpox was half way through the sixth century AD. It was prevalent throughout the Middle East and there is good documentation of several Calephs in Arabia dying of the disease. There is no clear evidence of it invading Europe at this time, but it seems highly probable that it did. Epidemics described by Marius of Avenches and Gregory of Tours in the sixth century AD and by Bede in England in the seventh century AD were probably smallpox (Creighton, 1891). A remarkably accurate clinical description of smallpox is given by the Persian physician Abu El Razi Rhazes (AD 860–932). The disease appears to have been prevalent throughout Europe during the Middle Ages. Its entry into Central America and Mexico is recorded in the sixteenth century AD. An invasion of the smallpox virus which occurred in the sixth century AD established a terrestrial reservoir which has been maintained almost up to the present day. Epidemic outbreaks have occurred sporadically in many parts of the world, and the disease has remained endemic throughout this period in a few localised parts of the world.

Quarantine measures which have been rigorously enforced during the past couple of decades combined with an intensive vaccination programme have now made the disease virtually extinct. The World Health Organisation has recently declared the world smallpox-free, except for a very localised area in Ethiopia. It seems most likely that smallpox will soon be eradicated from Ethiopia too. A major victory against one of man's deadliest enemies would then have been won. But the story of successive visitations of smallpox spaced several hundreds of years apart is perhaps a warning against excessive complacency. The evidence clearly points to smallpox coming from a cometary source. Because of the long-lasting property of the virus itself, and because of the high infectivity of the disease, a reservoir which lasts for some centuries is established on Earth. Then follows a long period when smallpox is extinct, then a further arrival of the virus, a further reservoir, and so on.

We have so far looked at a number of diseases which are present today and which are known to have existed in the past. We have traced the history of these diseases either indirectly through literary allusions or directly in medical writings. There is also the possibility that many ancient diseases existed which are now extinct. The Plague of Athens which we discussed in Chapter 2 is an example of such a disease. The English Sweats of the Middle Ages may have been a particularly virulent form of the influenza virus, but if it was so, it was of a type which has never since returned.

The prospect of new disease taking us unawares is depressing. Yet it is a possibility that is nonetheless real and it cannot be ignored. The theory discussed in this book leads us to expect a pattern of infectious disease which changes with time. We have seen that such changes occurred in the past and we may expect similar changes in the future, including the advent of new diseases from time to time.

In July 1976 an American Legion Convention which was held in Philadelphia had an unwelcome visitation. There was a highly localised epidemic of acute respiratory disease of a most unusual sort. From a total of 3,683 convention delegates and attendees, 183 were attacked, and there were 29 deaths. The victims spanned a wide age range. The onset of the severe symptoms of the disease was preceded by a day of malaise and muscle pain. This was followed by a rapidly rising fever to a very high maximum with rigours, cough, chest pain and difficulty in breathing. The course of the disease was swift and unpredictable. The death rate was high and antibiotics were found to be ineffective in the main. After an intensive laboratory search, a bacillus of variable length was identified in January 1977 as the causative agent. Subsequently it was found that antibodies specific to this bacillus were present in blood sera that were collected as far back as 1947. The implication is that this disease was present in the human population for some time, perhaps in a clinically less virulent form. But there were many fundamental questions that remained unanswered. Where did the bacillus come from? How is the disease transmitted? If it is infectious, why did none of the doctors and nurses attending the victims contract the disease?

Careful enquiries revealed that all those who were attacked spent a long time in a certain hotel lobby. There appears to have been a connection between the attack rate of the disease and the time spent on a pavement outside the hotel watching a parade. A distinction could even be made between those who were on opposite sides of the street. There is a strong indication of an airborne pathogen, the incidence of which was patchy on the scale of the width of the street.

Following the Philadelphia attack in 1976, Legionnaires' disease has appeared sporadically in several American states, and it has also made an entry into Europe and Britain. The individual cases, or clusters of cases, are normally so diffusely distributed that the usual theories of disease propagation involving the maintenance of a reservoir and transmission from person to person face sever difficulties.

9

Disease Against Mankind

Most people find the learning of mathematics difficult and boring, and it is not hard to understand why. In mathematical text everything is ordered like a tape-recording. Perhaps the best-known mathematical tape-recording is the geometry of Euclid, where every little bit of it must be there and always in the same place, otherwise the whole structure of the argument loses its meaning and validity. Yet among real mathematicians it is quite otherwise. Real mathematicians are perpetually seeing connections between diverse aspects of mathematics, a bit of algebra here, a pinch of geometry there, a remark on complex variable, a sudden flash of functional analysis. The thinking of real mathematicians is a complex multi-dimensional affair. The tape-recordings which students are required to wade through separately and sequentially have all become woven together into a kind of intellectual Jacob's coat, whose wearing is by no means a bore.

It is the same with music, although to begin with in early life the tape-recordings which constitute the great sonatas and symphonies have a brighter sheen to them than a Euclid text. But in later life, one becomes aware that every bar of the music is always preceded by exactly the same bar, and it is always followed by exactly the same bar. How one longs for the great composers themselves to be back on the scene to stir things up a bit.

There is abroad in the world a tape-recording still more restrictive than anything which mathematics or music imposes on us. This is the tape-recording of life itself. We are all condemned to go through life individual bar by individual bar. Older people who remember how Harold Larwood's bowling on the meticulously-prepared plumb wickets of the early 1930s terrorised the batsmen of his day can hardly help believing he would have made a farce out of modern cricket. Yet it is impossible to be certain because the bit of the tape-recording with Harold Larwood in it can never be snipped out and played alongside the bit that constitutes modern cricket. More the pity, for think of the crowd that would turn out to watch Larwood in his prime moving up to bowl on a fast wicket at Lord's against Mr Packer's World XI. Think of the roar of the crowd watching Ty Cobb play in a modern World Series. And the literary world too would have its interesting mixing of snippets from the tape-recording of life. A Proust or a Kafka, to say nothing of a D. H. Lawrence or a Virginia Woolf, can hardly have help wondering how marriage between Gustave Flauber and Emily Brontë would have turned out.

Comparing different portions of the tape-recording of life, however, is not entirely a matter of speculation and idle amusement. We are not complete prisoners entombed within our own time capsule, flicked away from the centre of the stage as

The Moving Finger writes; and,
    having writ,
Moves on; …

There are certain specially chosen bits of history that can be set alongside each other with a tolerable measure of objectivity. Military performance is an interesting example. We know the weapons and their capabilities in various ages, we know the number of men deployed on the battlefield in those various ages, we know the tactics employed by the commanders. With the reasonable assumption that men in one age were about equally as strong, brave or otherwise, intelligent or otherwise, as in another age, it is possible to match the different portions of the military tape-recording of history in a meaningful way. How would Alexander's army at Gaugamela in 331 BC have fared against Henry V at Agincourt in AD 1415? Questions like this become susceptible of an answer.

We suspect it to be axiomatic with most military theoreticians that in such comparisons the later army is thought to have been always the stronger. In each individual battle the stronger side wins. And since battles are going on almost perpetually there must be, one might suppose, a selective evolution towards greater and greater military power. How else could it be? Yet was Henry V really stronger than Alexander the Great? The answer is, of course, an emphatic no. Henry's army was but a miserable immobile skirmishing party that Alexander would not even have deigned to face himself, but would have expected any of a score of subordinates to have dispatched as easily as brushing aside a fly on a summer's day.

Doubtless there will be persons who never take a positive statement like this on trust, persons who would continue to argue, even as the snow closed over their heads, that an avalanche was not really bearing down upon them, persons who would in this case maintain that Henry's archers were better than Alexander's. The longbow, it might be said, had a greater range than the bows used by classical armies. So could Henry not have dug himself in, and then simply have held Alexander off for as long as he wanted? The answer once again is an emphatic no. The longbow had a range of about 200 yards. Against a sitting duck, such as Henry and his army would have been, Alexander had weapons of much greater range, weapons designed specifically to prevent such a digging in by a recalcitrant enemy.

Alexander is known to have placed great reliance on stone catapults. With the thought of modern artillery in our minds, we are apt to smile at such devices. Yet actual trials with reconstructed catapults have shown them to be capable of a surprisingly effective performance. The motive power, obtained by torsion applied to animal sinew or to women's hair, was sufficient to propel a ball of stone weighing up to 10 lb. at a speed of more than 200 ft per second, sufficient for a missile ejected at an elevation angle of 45° to have a horizontal range of about 500 yards. A stone ball would splinter naturally in the manner of shrapnel on hard impact, giving a much greater target area than an arrow. Digging himself in, with only the longbow for defence, would have been quite suicidal for Henry V.

At Gaugamela, on the plain near the ruins of ancient Nineveh, Alexander deployed 40,000 foot soldiers and 7000 cavalry. The Greek army was highly professional, with long training in the art of rapid and complex manoeuvre. The Persian army is said, probably with some exaggeration, to have numbered 200,000. The Persians were defeated by a successful Greek deception on the right wing, where Alexander began the engagement with a carefully stacked disposition of fast-moving cavalry. At Agincourt, King Henry had 5000 men, with only a small fraction of them mounted on cart-horses. The main English army took up a fixed position within a stockade of pointed stakes driven into the ground. The French army numbered about 25,000, and it is hard to conceive of any way in which it could have been defeated by its smaller, essentially static opponent. Yet the French commander managed to find a way. The mounted French, greatly outnumbering the mounted English, urged their own carthorses insistently into the English thickets of pointed stakes, which naturally penetrated the unprotected underbellies of the animals (perhaps suggesting to Winston Churchill his wartime phrase 'the soft underbelly of the Axis'). The armoured French were toppled from their wounded horses, and being heavily encumbered were unable to rise to their feet, and so were dispatched as they lay helplessly on the ground, like so many beetles turned over on their backs. If we could displace snippets from the tape-recording of time, it would be interesting in AD 1415, nearly seventeen and a half centuries after Gaugamela, to have had the great Alexander there as a spectator, watching the astonishingly inept scene that unfolded on the battlefield at Agincourt. It would have been difficult to convince him that later armies are always superior to earlier ones.

The explanation of why classical armies were greatly superior to medieval ones lies of course in disease, with which the medieval age was riddled. Classical times were comparatively disease-free, although ironically Alexander himself was hit by disease, probably of the low-latitude insect-borne variety, rather than one of the air-borne varieties of Europe and the Mediterranean. From the point of view of disease, the far-flung conquests of Alexander seem at first sight to have a foolhardy look about them, but they become more understandable when we consider that Alexander and his officers were almost certainly not used to thinking of disease as a serious factor. In contrast, disease in medieval Europe prevented an army of 25,000, such as the French deployed at Agincourt, from being anything other than a disorganised rabble, for the reason that a number as large as 25,000 could not be held together for long enough to turn them into an effective fighting unit. Medieval disease held down the largest armies that could be maintained at a professional level to mere fractions of the impressively large armies of classical times. Henry V won at Agincourt because his army was nearer to optimum size for the conditions of his day than was the French army.

The traveller who visits the ruined Roman villas on the Palatine Hill, the spaciously laid-out buildings of Pompeii, the open-air theatre with a seating capacity for some 20,000 persons at Epidaurus in the north-eastern Peloponnese, and who compares these relics of classical times with the medieval towns of Europe, with their castles on local hills above small clusters of hovels, will understand the crucial difference between a disease-free and a disease-riddled society.

Historical studies give us no very explicit answer to why the quality of medieval life should have been so much poorer than that of ancient Greece and Rome. We read of 'decline and fall' in the sense of Edward Gibbon, as if to imply that some inner understanding had become lost. But understanding in an objectively defined sense had certainly not become lost. Indeed quite the reverse. A reading of the massive volumes of *The History of Technology* (Oxford, 1957) shows that, except in the fine arts, the ability to cope with practical problems was unquestionably superior in medieval times. There have been no marked ups and downs in the history of technology — it has been upwards all the way, at any rate over the past 10,000 years.

Faced with this seeming contradiction, there have in recent years been attempts to explain the decline of Rome in less vaguely psychological terms. One suggestion is that the aristocratic classes were inadvertently poisoned by the lead pipes used to carry drinking water. We think this a poor suggestion. Alternatively, economic issues have been raised, such as the suggestion that there was too much olive-growing in Italy, with too much consequent reliance on grain supplies imported from abroad. Again we think this a weak argument. Then of course we have the barbarian assault from the east, the explanation so much favoured in older texts. But the barbarian assaults of the fourth and fifth centuries were not in the least new. From its earliest days, Rome had experienced barbarian invasions, some at least as formidable as those of the fifth century.

In the previous chapter we mentioned Galen's descriptions of what were at that time apparently new diseases (although they had probably been present in Egypt fifteen hundred years earlier). This, in our view, was the beginning of a disease-filled epoch, mounting in its intensity in succeeding centuries, to the Plague of Justinian in the sixth century, and continuing with devastating smallpox epidemics in the sixth and seventh centuries. It was this disease-riddled epoch that in our view caused the decline of Rome, and which brought about the onset of the Dark Ages. Disease forced humans to disperse, to move further apart on the average from each other, to uncivilise themselves.

We also attribute the rise of Christianity to the same disease-filled epoch. The older boisterous religions of Greece and Rome were excellent for healthy peoples, but they came to seem inappropriate in more sombre times. Nor is it an accident that the most sombre of all religions, Judaism, came in the thirteenth century BC out of disease-riddled Egypt. The Biblical account of Moses and the Hebrews (Hebrew in Egyptian means 'artisan') lays emphasis, correctly we think, on disease being the cause of the inability of the Pharaoh to prevent the Exodus (i.e. the loss of a major component of the Egyptian work-force). Likely enough, the Biblical account refers to the end of the Nineteenth Dynasty, which less than a century earlier had been represented by powerful rulers, Ramses I and Seti I.

It seems clear that the advance of technology over the disease-filled millennium from about AD 400 to AD 1400 provided the springboard for the almost explosive emergence of modern society. Throughout this millennium disease prevented technological discoveries from being fully exploited, in part objectively by preventing the growth of major population centres, and in part through the rigid dogmatism of a morose and intolerant religion. Nothing in the way of a spirited development of society could take place, no matter how extensive the increase in technical ability and understanding. Slowly, however, the shackles were cut away through the fifteenth and sixteenth centuries, so that by the seventeenth century Europe was poised to make the irresistible thrust which at last re-established something of the spontaneity and the intellectual quality of the age of classical Greece.

Our modern society is currently much more fortunate in its ability to cope with disease. Nowadays we are relatively disease-free, in the sense that the diseases now being driven most strongly from space, influenza and the common cold, happen to be comparatively innocuous. A diseased-epoch would be one in which the opposite situation held, with driven diseases the serious ones, like smallpox and bubonic plague.

What of the future? Our view must be less optimistic than that of the World Health Organisation, or the Health, Education, and Welfare Department of the US Government, which raises enormous taxes each year by promising a similarly comforting future to Americans. The day will assuredly come when appalling diseases will once again incident upon us from outside space. One hopes that this day is still many centuries away. When it eventually comes, medical science in alliance with the physical sciences will not again be in the helpless posture that Thucydides described in his account of the disease of 430 BC, nor again in the wretched state of mind of the fourteenth century when the best judgement medical opinion could offer for the cause of the Black Death was that it constituted a punishment from God.

The long evolution of animals on the Earth appears to have established the fortunate rule that the more virulent the attack of a pathogen the greater is our immunity response to it. The existence of a strong immunity response opens the way to the use of protective vaccines. This is because a strong response can be triggered by a deliberately induced pathogenic attack that is far milder than the main disease itself, as for instance in the use of a deliberately provoked attack of cowpox as a defence against the much more serious disease of smallpox. Since it takes months and perhaps even years for micrometeorites to settle down through the stratosphere, there will be time available for the development of such vaccines. We think the day will come when the upper atmosphere will be patrolled routinely for the incidence of pathogenic invaders from space.

The thoughtfully religious person who has read to this point will not have passed our reference to 'a morose and intolerant religion' without misgivings, and perhaps not without the question: What better have you people to offer in the way of an understanding of the meaning of life? Nothing of a panacea. If there were a panacea with any quality to it, then surely we would all know of it already. A small chink in the curtain perhaps, opening up on still quite unknown territory. We end this chapter with speculations that will serve to introduce the next chapter.

Watch a vivisectionist at work. Then imagine yourself in the position of the animal victim. So it is with all of us. We are all the victims of an enormous vivisectionist experiment. In one respect 'our' vivisectionist is similar to a human vivisectionist, and in another respect 'He' is different. 'He' is different in possessing the qualities of what, for the want of a better word, we call a superintellect. 'He' is the same in not being in the least degree squeamish about the experiment. A squeamish 'He' would not have permitted disease and suffering, as many centuries ago St Augustine was quick to notice.* In our final chapters we shall explain why, in the way things are, there *had* to be disease and suffering. The

*Having posed a great problem correctly, St Augustine was then forced off into a flaccid backwater in attempting to solve it. St Augustine lived, unfortunately, in the wrong bit of the tape-recording of life.

concept is a little unusual. 'Good' is the desired end of the experiment. But it is not permitted, even by 'God', to achieve 'good' through arbitrary decrees, as is usually supposed in religious thought. 'Good' must be achieved through complete intellectual and logical rigour. Only through rigour is there a reliable sanity in the 'experiment'. This appears to be the overwhelming message of biology, as we shall come to see it in our remaining chapters.

10

Viruses and Evolution

In this penultimate chapter we shall consider how the acquisition of viruses from space may well be related to the evolution of plants and animals here on the Earth. The higher plants and animals carry a heredity with some one million genes, represented in detail by a 1000 million or more base-pairs arranged like ties along a rail track. The rails are not straight and parallel but are twisted into the Crick–Watson double helix. Presumably for convenience in packing within the living cell, the double helix is chopped into pieces, chromosomes, which number 46 in man — a typical number for higher plants and animals.

There are four kinds of base-pair, which we can think of simply as P, Q, R, S, and it is through the use of P, Q, R, S that the message of heredity is conveyed. A language provided with only four letters would obviously be very restricted, and biology copes with this problem by combining the base-pairs three-at-a-time to give 64 triplets of base-pairs (4 choices for the first base-pair, 4 for the second, and 4 for the third, giving a total of $4 \times 4 \times 4 = 64$ distinct triplets). However, the resulting 64 letters (a 'letter' now being a triplet of base-pairs) apparently provided too rich a situation, so that the number of effective letters has been cut down to 20, by treating several triplets as the same letter. The third base-pair in the triplets plays the main role in this redundancy, with say PQR and PQQ treated as the same letter. Sometimes too the third base-pair plays no role at all, with say RSP, RSQ, RSR, RSS all treated for the purposes of heredity as the same letter. This redundancy situation suggests that the letters were originally made up of only two base-pairs, with $4 \times 4 = 16$ possibilities. The 16 possibilities of the form

PQ proved insufficient, however, so the third base-pair was tacked on. But the resulting jump from only 16 letters to 64 proved too big a step, so the redundancies were introduced to keep the number of letters down to a manageable number, i.e. to 20.

With only 20 letters needed out of 64 possibilities, some of the triplets became available for use as marks to indicate the beginnings and endings of words. While the number of letters used in the alphabet of heredity is comparable with the number used in an actual language, 20 for heredity compared to the 26 letters of the English alphabet, the words of heredity are enormously long compared to the words of ordinary language. Heredity words almost always contain more than a hundred letters, and some words may even contain more than a thousand letters. In ordinary language, long words have sharply defined meanings whereas short words are normally used in several different ways. Thus the words 'solitude' and 'uncompromising' have unmistakable meanings, whereas 'by', 'for', 'to' and 'the' tell us little or nothing by themselves. So it need not surprise us that the 'words' of heredity, with their enormous lengths, carry a great deal of precise meaning, to a point where heredity has no need for paragraphs. The words are veritable paragraphs in themselves.

Just as the words of ordinary language can be related to provide special meanings, so several heredity words are often related to each other. Ordinary words are sometimes combined in ways that retain something of their individual meanings, as for instance in 'present-day'. 'Present-day', however, has a meaning beyond the literal day that we are experiencing now. If we were comparing medieval industry with present-day industry, we might well mean by 'present-day' a time span of a few decades. Ordinary words are also sometimes strung together into idioms with meanings quite different from anything implied by the individual words themselves. Thus 'pie in the sky' scarcely ever involves a pie, and even if it did the pie would certainly not be up in the sky. Heredity words are often strung together in similar ways, and some biologists prefer to think in terms of these word associations as the basic units of heredity, calling them 'genes'. In this way of looking at the situation the individual words are called 'cistrons'. Others prefer to equate 'gene' with cistron, which is the practice we shall adopt in this chapter. A gene therefore represents a sequence of triplets of base-pairs, going from a particular mark at the beginning of a word to a mark at the end. (For a more detailed discussion of such markings see Appendix 3.)

It is with this definition that we now return to the opening statement of this chapter, that the chromosomes of higher plants and animals carry approximately a million genes. If we go a long way back into the past, say a 1000 million years ago, we arrive at much more primitive forms with far less than a million genes in their genetic material. The higher plants and animals must therefore have acquired genes at an average rate of about one new gene per thousand years. During exceptionally rapid periods of evolution, as for instance in the emergence of the mammals over the past 50 million years, the rate of acquisition of new genes must have been considerably faster than this average rate. During rapid periods of evolution the rate must at least have been one new gene acquired every few centuries. The question we now have to ask is where the new genes came from.

The answer proposed in this chapter is that the new genes came from the acquisition of viruses which joined themselves to the genetic material of plants and animals, the viruses themselves coming from space. This means that biological evolution has been largely dictated by the addition of new heritable material from space, not through continuing small modifications of existing material. We can even imagine the occasional addition of a whole bacterium, perhaps resulting in an increase, not just of the number of genes, but of the number of the chromosomes of plants and animals.

The first encouragement to this idea comes from the study of the past history of plants and animals, particularly with respect to rates of evolutionary change. These indicate that the big steps in evolution occur in jumps, often sudden jumps from species to species (see for example a review of Thomas J. M. Schopf, 'Patterns of Evolution: A Summary and Discussion', appearing as Chapter 17 in *Patterns of Evolution as Illustrated by the Fossil Record*, Elsevier

Scientific, 1977, ed. A. Hallam). The small mutational steps of Mendelian heritable change are not well-suited to the understanding of such major jumps, whereas the sudden incorporation of a substantial new block of genetic material, such as the addition of an entire bacterium, would seem to provide for a better understanding of the situation.

From a broad biological point of view this means that the invasion of the Earth by viruses and bacteria from space is a crucially necessary phenomenon. As individuals we tend to see things differently, of course, since such invasions threaten our health and perhaps even our lives. But it is characteristic of biological evolution that it rarely serves the interest of the individual. Indeed it is by ruthlessly discarding unwanted individuals that evolution proceeds. This suffering of diseases by individuals would be of no consequence at all, so long as some survived, and so long as new genetic material continued to be acquired.

At this point it will be as well to discuss the nature of viruses in a little more detail than we have done hitherto. In the following passage Sir Christopher Andrewes described the invasion of a cell by a virus particle, with particular reference to a rhinovirus, a type which produces the common cold. (*The Common Cold*, Weidenfeld and Nicolson, London, 1965, page 23.)

> A virus consists essentially of a coil of a very complicated organic chemical, nucleic acid, which carries with it all the information, the specifications, necessary for making more virus of the same sort. Knowledge is rapidly being gained nowadays, as to how a chemical substance can carry instructions to the cell to carry out certain chemical synthetic processes. The molecules strung along the nucleic acid thread seem to act as a sort of mould or template, and other molecules are assembled in contact with this thread to make another elongated structure; the molecules of which are strung together in a very precise manner. Associated with the nucleic acid is protein, a primary function of which seem to be to protect the precious nucleic acid from being destroyed by hostile chemical substances in its environment. Another function is probably to make specific contact with the cell to be infected. The

protein may be wrapped round the nucleic acid in spiral manner, as in the influenza virus, or it may be packed around it in a number of similar components to form a regular crystal-like twenty-sided figure. This is what poliomyelitis and probably rhinoviruses also look like, and they are just about the smallest viruses known.

What happens when a virus infects a cell is probably something like this. The protein part of a virus makes specific contact with something on the cell-surface. Then the cell ingests or takes the virus up within itself. It may ingest the whole virus and break it up inside or, as happens with the bacteriophages or viruses infecting bacteria, the protein coat of the virus may be left outside the cell, only the essential nucleic acid gaining access to the interior. In either event, the protein part of the virus is expendable and plays no further part. The nucleic acid part, however, proceeds to instruct the cellular mechanism in a sinister manner. Suppose it is a rhinovirus infecting a cell lining your nose. The instruction will run thus: 'Stop making the ingredients necessary for making more nose-cells. Henceforth use your chemical laboratory facilities for making more nucleic acid like me.' The intruding virus nucleic acid gives the further instruction: 'And now make a lot of protein of such-and-such composition which I require wherewith to coat myself.' The cell can do nothing but obey and as more new virus particles are thus assembled by the cell's chemical mechanisms they are, at the end of the production-line, turned out into the outside of the cell. With many viruses, including probably rhinoviruses, the final effect is to exhaust the cell altogether, so that after a while it dies and disintegrates. The virus set free will infect more of its victim's cells until such time as defence mechanisms have been mobilised. It will also get into the outside world and infect more victims, for one result of the cell-destruction in the course of a cold infection will be inflammation, pouring out of fluid, sneezing and spread of virus. All of it a very conveniently organised affair for the benefit of rhinoviruses.

This may be true of the rhinovirus, yet other viruses have the well-proven ability in some cases of not destroying host cells but of developing a symbiotic relation with them. In some such cases the viral genetic material is actually known to add itself to the host genetic material, inevitably contributing several new genes at one fell swoop. So the process we are discussing quite certainly exists. What presumably happens is that a species which is persistently attacked over a long period by a particular virus gradually develops immunity to that virus, which is then forced into an increasingly passive role, to be eventually restricted in its multiplication to the natural division of the cell itself — in other words it multiplies only with the cell, like all other genetic material.

The detailed discussion of Appendix 3 shows that the purely terrestrial development of significantly new genes cannot have occurred at anything approaching a rate of 1 per 1000 years. Accepting that the numbers of non-repetitive genes are only changed in an important degree by extraterrestrial effects, we can see how a difficulty that for long tormented the nineteenth-century geologist Charles Lyell (and which even Darwin himself found unanswerable) can now be cleared up. Lyell believed deeply in the long-term constancy of the terrestrial environment, a belief which modern geology has fully vindicated, at any rate for the past 1000 million years. Lyell therefore argued that if the environment has had long-term constancy, then so must terrestrial life forms. This follows inevitably from Darwinian evolution, which optimises plants and animals to their environment. So if the environment is unchanging, so must be the plants and animals. The one condition must imply the other. Yet paleontologists of the early nineteenth century argued that the fossil record showed otherwise, to which Lyell replied that the fossil record — incomplete in his own day — would eventually turn out to support the long-term constancy of biological forms. So far as the vertebrates are concerned this constancy has not existed, and the evolutionary dilemma seen so clearly by Lyell, and admitted by Darwin, remains with us to this day. What, we may ask, has brought about the undoubtedly increasing complexity of the paleontological record? Our answer is the increasing aggregate of cometary genes, against which terrestrial natural selection has been able to operate. What we are saying now is that biological evolution is subject to an external control of heritable materials, and as this changes so do the optimum life forms produced by Darwinian selection.

Some microbiologists have been worried about the concept of diseases coming from space, because it seemed to them that the relation between the chemical systems of terrestrial cells and the invading viruses from space was too intimate. How could the invaders know about the cells they would encounter on reaching the Earth? How could viruses have their mode of attack prepared in advance as precisely as the above quotation from Sir Christopher Andrewes shows to be the case? The answer is that the terrestrial cells to be attacked were their kind of stuff, built with their kind of chemical logic. Furthermore, the genetic material of terrestrial creatures, is itself a conglomeration of viruses and bacteria, and viruses and bacteria had already learned to prey on each other — the viruses breaking up the bacteria, and the bacteria incorporating and swallowing up the viruses into themselves — all this taking place within their cometary homes. What happens here on Earth is only an extension of what happened before, an extension to a different physical environment with different selective pressures, but not with a different system of biochemistry.

There are many general arguments to show that this view of the situation is correct. Otherwise is it not remarkable, within the usual Earth-bound theories of biological evolution and of the indigenous nature of bacteria and viruses, that complex terrestrial life forms have failed during their long history to develop a total immunity to all infectious diseases? One almost has to argue in attempting to answer this question that pathogens can 'think', in the sense of being able to accommodate themselves to every immunological device which their hosts may adopt. But of course, bacteria and viruses possess no such literal ability. They can only evolve in a Darwinian sense in relation to the immunities developed by their hosts. If a host should happen to possess a form of immunity for which no answering mutation were in existence, there is no intellectual sense in which a pathogen could set about inventing such a mutation. Pathogens must always have already in hand mutations for dealing with the immunological shifts of their hosts, otherwise they become extinct. Pathogens are thus balanced on razor edge between survival and extinction, a balance which seems to us to be more acceptable if it has only to be maintained on time-scales of centuries or millennia, rather than for the much longer time-scales that must necessarily be involved in an Earth-bound theory.

Virulent viruses are particularly exposed to extinction. There are four steps in the complex process whereby such a virus multiplies itself, the preventing of any one of which would confer immunity on an evolved plant or animal. The virus must first have an attachment protein fitted to an attachment site on the wall of a host cell. Second, the interaction of the attachment protein to the cell wall must serve eventually to strip other viral proteins away from the genetic material of the virus, which must then be afforded naked ingress to the host cell. Third, the viral genetic material must have the ability to overwrite the normal genetic programme of the cell. And fourth, after multiplying in number, the new virus particles must be able to gain egress from the host cell in order to attack new cells.

With so many opportunities to frustrate the attack of viruses, and yet with evolved life forms failing to avail themselves convincingly of these opportunities, we have — within the Earth-bound point of view — the making of a contradiction. Immunity, such as it is, consists mostly of preventing the entry of virus particles, and then only the entry of specific viruses, not of viruses in general. It would be far more effective for host cells to develop genetically so as to prevent overwriting by viruses in general. Logically, such a process must exist, because the great quantity of information present in the genetic material of the host must be able to overcome the combined information of many viruses. Yet such a defence is never presented, except possibly very transiently during the course of an infection, when a substance called 'interferon' may have some such effect. The more likely explanation is that host cells deliberately avoid the apparently best form of defence. The situation is not at all that the virus is 'clever' but that the host appears to be incorrigibly stupid.

Indeed host cells even seem to invite the invasion of viruses by deliberately providing sites to which viruses can attach themselves.

The contradiction we have just outlined, which has also been noticed by N. G. Anderson, *Nature*, 227, 1347 (1970), disappears of course as soon as we turn from the Earth-bound point of view to the incidence of viruses and bacteria from outside the Earth, and consider this incidence as being an essential and crucial requirement for biological evolution to occur here. Terrestrial plants and animals could not then develop immunity to pathogenic attack, since to do so would be to preclude the addition of further genes to themselves. Failure to adapt to an ever-changing environment would then ensue, with the inevitable consequence that such an immune life form would soon fail to match the competition from other non-immune forms. The immune form would become extinct.

Viruses differ markedly among themselves. They differ in size, from the small picornaviruses, no more than about a millionth of a centimetre in diameter, up to the complex poxviruses with dimensions some ten times larger. Viruses also differ considerably in the biochemical structure of their genetic material, and greatly too in their geometrical shapes. Some thirty types have been recognised, and the question of whether these many types could have had a common ancestor has been raised. Could the larger viruses, for example, be the forerunners of the smaller ones? The lack of any known intermediate forms indicates negative answers to these questions. More significantly, it would be difficult to connect continuously in an evolutionary scheme the different geometrical forms, particularly the precise structures of icosahedral patterns. It is therefore likely that the different types of virus are distinct from each other, as we would expect if they were derived from different cometary homes. But all have an interaction with the cells of terrestrial life forms, because the latter are conglomerates built by genetic accretions from many cometary sources. Terrestrial life forms are therefore integrations over the whole of the invading army of viruses and bacteria.

The view that viruses originate through the breakdown and degeneration of cells was popularly held some years ago. This view, which is less in favour today than it used to be, would be opposed to the present theory. Instead of accretion of viruses into cells, one would have the breakdown of cells into viruses. The problem with this older idea is to understand how the cells of the higher animals could have acquired new genetic material at an average rate of one gene in every few centuries. This difficulty will be seen all the more clearly when we come in Appendix 3 to consider the rate at which base-pair triplets of genetic material can undergo changes by random mutation.

There is, however, a class of virus of approximately spherical shape, the type-C viruses, which are indeed intrinsically generated by cells. The type-C viruses appear to be genes carried by the genetic material of reptiles, birds and mammals. Breakdown occurs in the body cells, with the type-C viruses emerging and multiplying rather in the manner of tumour-causing viruses. The latter are sometimes acquired from outside, whereas the similar type-C viruses are generated from within an animal.

The production of type-C viruses can also be inhibited. They exist in profusion within the fetal placenta of mammals, but become suppressed shortly before birth. It seems that the transfer of these viruses into genetic material is a two-way process. The virus can be incorporated into genetic material, and it can also break loose and free itself from the cell. This it may do as an animal ages, or after a number of generations have intervened. The view has grown strongly in recent years that the spontaneous break-loose of type-C viruses within animals is the principal cause of cancers, and therefore the research in this field — much of it at the National Cancer Institute, Bethesda, Maryland — has been carried on intensively.[*]

Type-C viruses are particularly relevant to this discussion because one such virus has been discovered in the great cats and baboons of the old world, but not in baboons of the new world.

---

[*]G. J. Todaro & R. J. Huenber, *Proc. Nat. Acad. USA*, 69, 1009, 1972.
R. R. Benveniste *et al.*, *Nature*, 248, 17, 1974.
C. J. Sherr *et al.*, *Proc. Nat. Acad. Sc. USA*, 71, 3721, 1974.

The possession of the genetic material giving rise to this virus is therefore a matter of geography not of speciation. We have seen in former chapters that epidemics of disease have geographical foci. The foci are often less than continental in scale, and indeed in the case of influenza the incidence is patchy in extreme detail. We can therefore conceive of a virus being incorporated into genetic material at one geographical site, but not at other sites. The incorporation will then gradually become spread from the initial site to the extent to which animals can move out from that site. In the case of animals in the old world, the spread is through the old world itself, not across the deep ocean to the new world.

11
Diseases from Space

In this final chapter we begin with a brief synopsis and reappraisal of our main arguments. The starting point of our argument was based upon four observations:

(1) The interstellar clouds of gas and dust contain vast quantities of organic materials. Such materials were added to the outer regions of the solar system over tens of millions of years following the formation of the solar system itself.

(2) Material on the outside of the solar system took several hundreds of millions of years to form the planets Uranus and Neptune, and during this long time-interval the condensed bodies were cometary objects, many billions of them. Indeed a considerable fraction of the objects survived to the present day. A vast swarm of comets still exists as a great halo surrounding the solar system. The proportions of the main life-forming elements in comets — hydrogen, carbon, nitrogen and oxygen — are uncannily similar to the proportions found in living material. The total quantity of these principal life-forming elements contained in the whole halo of present-day comets could be as much as ten times the mass of the whole Earth.

(3) Conditions on the primitive Earth were not at all favourable for the origin of life to have occurred here. The likely presence of oxygen in the early terrestrial atmosphere would soon have destroyed any organic molecules which happened to be present here. In comets, however, the conditions were highly favourable for the origin of life. Liquid solutions involving water, hydrogen cyanide, hydrogen sulphide and many organic molecules from

interstellar space were safely buried here under a few hundred metres of surface skin. For a single comet, the volume of such a liquid solution was of the order of ten thousand cubic kilometres. There were billions of comets with such solutions, each with sufficient chemical energy of its own to maintain a moderate internal temperature of, say, 10°C for millions of years.

(4) The orbits of individual comets in the swarm around the solar system are constantly fluctuating under the influence of the gravitational fields of the Sun, planets and passing stars. Occasionally a cometary orbit happens to be gravitationally perturbed in a way that brings it to the inner regions of the solar system, the regions of the planets Mercury, Venus, Earth and Mars. This invasion happens for about ten comets each year. During the few months that such a comet spends comparatively close to the Earth, the heating effect of the Sun causes evaporation of the outer layers, stripping the comet like peeling an onion skin by skin. The resulting emergence of gas and fine particles produces the visible coma and tail of a comet. Because of the continuing approach of a few comets each year to our vicinity, the Earth moves constantly through clouds of evaporated cometary material. Several hundred tons of this material are incident on the Earth's upper atmosphere each year. The material settles eventually to ground level.

Taking these four observations together, it is natural to suggest that the Earth received life from outside, through the entry into the upper atmosphere of living cell shed by comets. There is no requirement for the shedding process to have been efficient. The analogy of seeds blowing in the wind, with few destined to take root, comes readily to mind. It is sufficient for biological continuity that the few should survive. The safe arrival of even a few living cells would have carried the Earth across a huge chasm of bio-chemical, evolution, a chasm which would otherwise be well-nigh impossible to bridge.

Such a sequence of ideas might not have been too distasteful to orthodox opinion, which conventionally takes the Earth to be a closed system, except of course for sunlight, which enters from outside. The Earth, however, is manifestly not a closed system.

The vertical distance to the 'space' above our heads is not more than an hour's drive in a car (cf. Figure 2.1a). It is the Earth's gravitation that gives us the subjective impression of 'space' being very distant. Gravity is responsible for preventing us from moving easily upwards through the few tens of miles that would bring us to 'space'. For particles coming to us from space, however, gravity works the opposite way, by assisting downward motion into the atmosphere. From space to earth the connection is easy. If this connection were responsible only for the beginning of terrestrial life, with all subsequent developments proceeding according to evolution in a closed system here on the Earth, the price to be paid by orthodox opinion would not be very great, for little of existing biology would be changed.

Such a compromise between astronomy and biology would at first sight appear eminently reasonable. There was one further astronomical consideration, however, which did not permit us to accept this compromise as it stood. We noted above that the Earth moves constantly through evaporated cometary debris. If in the past such debris brought living cells to the Earth, it should still be doing so today. What was the evidence for or against this, conclusion?

We explained at the outset how our first thoughts were to suggest a search of cometary debris for bacteria and viruses, and of how we then came to realise that such a direct attack on the problem would not only be far more expensive than an epidemiological attack, but also quite probably much less sensitive. We were led therefore to the investigations discussed in previous chapters, and our own contribution was given in Chapter 6.

We have received many criticisms, some friendly, others less friendly, to the views we expressed in Chapter 6. The hostile criticism amounted to little beyond arguing that because we are not qualified medical practitioners, we have no business to be engaged in such matters. We mention this criticism in order to emphasise once again that not a single case among the more than twenty thousand school victims involved in our investigation was diagnosed by us. Our belief, from which we are not likely to be budged, is that school matrons and medical officers, with many year of practical experience, were able to diagnose influenza with sufficient precision for any few mistakes to have disappeared in the statistical analysis of the large number of cases contained in our survey. Apart from two or three returns to our questionnaire that were numerically ambiguous, and which we did not know how to interpret, all data involving influenza and no other disease were included in our analysis. If there had been any marked fluctuations in diagnostic standards, we could easily have seen them, as for instance in variations from school to school of the average number of days of class absence per victim. There were little or no such variations. We believe therefore that our survey was not only large in quantity but also uniform in quality, and we have the temerity to think that it will prove superior to others that may follow it on similar lines. Our reason for so thinking is that psychological factors, of which there are none at all in our survey, will inevitably arise once school authorities become aware in advance that an investigation is to be made.

Friendly critics of our view accept the findings of Chapter 6 and agree that influenza spreads by incidence from the air, not by person-to-person transmission. Granted this position, could the influenza virus not be sucked up into the air in one place and then deposited in other quite different places? The virus would need to become protected through some form of encapsulation, but — it is asked — why not? Certainly, the more one can invent an Earth-bound theory which simulates the cometary theory, the less we can object to it!

The concentration of the virus at distant places would surely be small compared to that at the home site. Yet the virus must nevertheless be highly infectious at distant places, in spite of its low concentration. To overcome this immediate difficulty, there would need to be a biosphere in which the virus could multiply and mutate while resident in the atmosphere. Birds as a vehicle of motion, multiplication and mutation come naturally to mind, but then there are the difficulties of the 1918–1919 winter epidemic in Alaska that we noted in Chapter 7. Birds apart, a biosphere existing in the upper atmosphere cannot be lightly dismissed and some technical argument is needed to assess this concept.

K. Nakajima, U. Desselberger and P. Palese have recently given interesting data (*Nature*, 274, 334, 1978) concerning the detailed genetic structure of H1 N1 (1977), obtained from the viral isolates of victims in the USSR and Hong Kong. The structure was found to be different from patient to patient, with respect to a number of places or 'spots' on the RNA of the virus, a 'spot' being a short sequence of bases on the ribose-phosphate strand of the RNA at well-defined locations (see Appendix 3). From an examination of about eight per cent of all the genes, about five such variations were found from one viral isolate to another, implying that there were differences of at least sixty bases for the whole of the genetic material.

We are doubtful, for reasons discussed in Appendix 3, that random copying errors involved in the simple multiplication of a virus could be responsible for this kind of situation. The many variations of base attachments in the viral RNA is indicative of enzymic repair following damage by ultraviolet light. Cometary debris in space could be nearly self-shielding. This could be achieved, for example, by particles travelling together in loosely bound aggregates, when only particles close to the surface of an aggregate would have damaging ultraviolet light incident upon them. Shock impact on entering the upper atmosphere, however, would cause such aggregates to fly apart into their constituent particles. While still above the ozone layer of the atmosphere, for a time of a few hours, a bacterium with a size of about 1 micron would be exposed to damage by ultraviolet light. The damage is of a kind that can often be repaired in ordinary sunlight by proteins (enzymes) contained within a bacterium. Several damaged virus particles within the same host cell can also pool their undamaged portions to produce a single new viable particle. When this happens, the new particle is different in its detailed structure from the old particles before they were damaged. Furthermore, restored particles never are quite the same, a fact which might well explain why the isolates of H1 N1 (1977) were different from one influenza victim to another.

A terrestrial atmospheric theory of virus dispersal can scarcely seek to imitate the cometary theory by appealing to ultraviolet light to explain the experimentally determined 'spot' variations, for it would be straining imagination too far to argue that virus particles were sucked up from ground level to altitudes above sixty kilometres, such as would be necessary to bring them well clear of the Earth's ozone layer, and so to give exposure to ultraviolet light at the appropriate wavelengths (2200 to 2800 Ångströms). The cometary theory contains the hazard of ultraviolet exposure, but the hazard has within it the advantageous possibility of explaining why influenza and the common cold virus are both capable of a vast number of variations. We consider that viral isolates from victims of these diseases may never be found to be genetically exactly the same, as indeed they have not been the same for the cases examined so far.

This brings us in conclusion to what appears a short proof of the correctness of the ideas of this book. We have just remarked on the highly efficient repair mechanisms which bacteria and viruses possess against damage by ultraviolet light with wavelengths around 2600 Ångströms. Yet bacteria and viruses at the Earth's surface do not experience this radiation naturally. Nor can they have done so according to orthodox theory, at any rate for several thousands of millions of years back into the past. To suppose that repair mechanisms would have been meticulously conserved in the absence of selective pressures to maintain them appears to us absurd. Indeed the proponents of the Earth-bound theory, when confronted by the epidemiologic facts of the preceding chapters, are likely to seek explanations of the facts by arguing that bacteria and viruses change at extraordinarily rapid rates, viruses in weeks or months, bacteria in years or centuries. One would think that the ability to adapt swiftly to the new would also imply the ability to slough off what had become unwanted — unwanted on a time scale, not merely of centuries, but of millions of centuries.

To explain the existence of repair mechanisms against damage by 2600 Ångströms radiation, it is usually argued that during the Earth's early history, when life is supposed to have originated, ultraviolet light at 2600 Ångströms penetrated the atmosphere. This situation occurred, it is supposed, before a shielding layer of atmospheric ozone was formed. There was then strong selective pressure for the evolution of ultraviolet repair mechanisms. If life existed in much its present biochemical form, there would certainly be selective pressure, but how could life exist in its present biochemical form in the presence of damaging ultraviolet *before* there were repair mechanisms? On a straightforward reckoning, this chicken-and-egg situation is self-contradictory, although we can imagine an edifice of further hypotheses that might permit the question to be answered in what is often described as 'hand-waving' style.

In our view, bacteria and viruses possess efficient ultraviolet repair mechanisms simply because without them they could not have made the journey safely from comet to Earth. The mechanisms evolved in the first place to permit the interchanges from comet to comet that we mentioned in Chapter 1, the universal process of shedding and seeding to which we attributed the biochemical unity of the solar system. Among the many billions of cometary laboratories, only a system that evolved towards immunity from radiation damage could have become a candidate for impressing itself as the master system for the solar system as a whole.

Bibliography

Chapter 1
F. Hoyle and N. C. Wickramasinghe, *Lifecloud*, Dent, London, 1978.

Chapter 2
C. G. A. Thomas, *Medical Microbiology*, London, 1973.
L. C. Hale, *Nature*, 268, 710, 1977.
Thucydides, *The Peloponnesian Wars*, translated by Benjamin Jowett.

Chapter 3
Hippocrates, *Ancient Medicine* (translated W. H. S. Jones), Penguin.
C. Andrewes, *The Common Cold*. Weidenfeld and Nicolson, London, 1965.
T. R. Allen, A. F. Bradburne, E. J. Scott, C. S. Goodwin and D. A. J. Tyrell, *Journal of Hygiene*, Cambridge, volume 71, 657, 1973.
M. Shibli, S. Gooch, H. E. Lewis and D. A. J. Tyrrell, *Journal of Hygiene*, Cambridge, 69, 255, 1971.
J. H. Paul and H. L. Freese, *American Journal of Hygiene*, 17, 517, 1933.
M. J. Holmes, T. R. Allen, A. F. Bradburne and E. J. Scott, *Journal of Hygiene*, Cambridge, 69, 194, 1971.
A. S. Cameron and B. W. Moore, *Journal of Hygiene*, Cambridge, 66, 427, 1968.

Chapter 4
W. I. B. Beveridge, *Influenza: The Last Great Plague*, Heinemann, London, 1977.
Influenza: Review of current Research, W. H. O. Monograph Series, 1952.
L. Weinstein, *New England Journal of Medicine*, 6 May 1976.
M. W. Paplan and R. G. Webster, *Scientific American*, December 1977.
C. Creighton, *A History of Epidemics in Great Britain*, Cambridge University Press, 1891.
The Lancet, 19 March, 1919.

Chapter 5

C. H. Stuart-Harris and G. C. Child, *Influenza*, E. Arnold, 1976.

P. Selby (ed.), *Influenza, Virus, Vaccines and Strategy*, Academic Press, 1976.

W. I. B. Beveridge, *ibid*.

J. Mulder and N. Masurel, *The Lancet*, i, 810, 1958.

S. J. Machen, C. W. Potter and J. S. Oxford, *Journal of Hygiene*, Cambridge, 68, 497, 1970.

Z. Sekanina, *Icarus*, 13, 475, 1970.

J. Mantle and D. A. J. Tyrrell, *Journal of Hygiene*, Cambridge, 71, 89, 1973.

R. H. Drachman, G. M. Hochbaum and I. M. Rosenstock, *Impact of Asian Influenza on Community Life: A Study in Five Cities*, Public Health Services Publication No. 766, 1960 (US Government Printing Office).

Chapter 6

F. Hoyle and N. C. Wickramasinghe, *New Scientist*, 28 April, 1978.

Chapter 7

Virgil (translated by K. R. Mackenzie), The Folio Society Limited, London, 1969.

Proceedings of the US Senate Committee On Appropriations, Washington DC.

Chapter 8

C. Creighton, *History of Epidemics in Great Britain*, Cambridge University Press, 1891.

J. K. Mitchell, *Trans. Ass. Amer. Phys.*, **15**, 134, 1900.

J. Moore, *History of the Smallpox*, Longmans, London, 1815.

D. Morse, D. R. Brothwell and P. J. Ucko, *Amer. Rev. Resp. Dis.*, 90, 524, 1964.

P. Razell, *New Scientist*, 20 October 1977.

Legionnaires Disease

J. E. McDade *et al.*, *New England Journal of Medicine*, 297, 1197, 1977.

V. W. Fraser *et al.*, *New England Journal of Medicine*, 297, 1189, 1977.

Poliomyelitis in isolated populations
T. H. Lewis and W. L. Brannon, *JAMA*, 230, 1295, 1974.
F. L. Black, JAMA, 232, 486, 1975.

Cholera
John Snow, 'The Broad Street Pump' in *Curiosities of Medicine*, ed. B. Rouéché, Brown & Co., 1963.
F. P. Smith, 'Smallpox in China', *Medical Times Gaz.*, ii, 277, 1871.
Charaka Samhita, translated by R. K. Sharma and V. B. Dash, Chowkhamba Sanskrit Series Office, Varanasi, India, 1976.
Sushruta Samhita, translated by K. K. L. Bhisagratan, 1907.
B. Ebbel, *The Papyrus Ebers*, Oxford University Press, London, 1937.
M. A. Roffer, *Studies in the Palaeopathology of Egypt*, Chicago University Press, Chicago, 1921.
L. F. Flick, *Development of our Knowledge of Tuberculosis*, Philadelphia, 1925.
M. A. Ruffer and A. R. Ferguson, *J. Path. Bact.*, 15, 1, 1911.
Hippocratic Writings (ed.) G. E. R. Lloyd, Pelican Classics, 1978.
Treatise on the Smallpox and Measles, Abu Beer Mohammed Ibn Zacariya Ar-Razi (commonly called RHAZES), translated by W. A. Greenhill, The Sydenham Soc., London, 1848.

Chapter 9
The History of Technology, Oxford University Press, 1957.

Chapter 10
A. Hallam (ed.) *Patterns of Evolution as Illustrated by the Fossil Record*, Elsevier, 1977.
N. G. Anderson, *Nature*, 227, 1347, 1970.
G. J. Todaro and R. J. Huenber, *Proc. Nat. Acad. USA*, 69, 1009, 1972.
R. R. Benvcniste *et al.*, *Nature*, 248, 17, 1974.
C. J. Sherr *et al.*, *Proc. Nat. Acad. USA*, 71, 3721, 1974.

Chapter 11
K. Nakajima, U. Desselberger and P. Palese, *Nature*, 274, 334, 1978.
T. R. G. Gray and J. R. Postgate, *The Survival of Vegetative Microbes*, Cambridge University Press, 1976.

Appendix 1
Organic Materials in Space

It is in general true that in all past ages, people suffered from wrong ideas about the nature of the world. Such ideas were passionately adhered to and defended at the time until eventually, with the advent of new facts, they came to be overturned. The same we believe to be true today in relation to all the "big ideas" about the physical world. One such big idea relates to the origin of life which in turn relates to the ideas of diseases and pandemics from space as are described in this book. The firm belief of many scientists is that life must necessarily be a purely terrestrial affair, and so also must all epidemics of diseases throughout recorded history. The first cell from which all the rest of life evolved, it is posited, arose as a result of chemicals coming together in some location on Earth — oceans, lakes, ponds or thermal vents — the canonical Aristotelean idea of spontaneous generation. Yet there is no hard evidence to support this belief. What is ignored or glossed over is the super-astronomically vast information content (in the form of the specific arrangements of relevant monomers) that is involved in even the simplest living cell.

The basic problem relating to the origin of life anywhere in the cosmos is to overcome a super-astronomical improbability hurdle that demands probabilistic resources that are certainly not available on the Earth [1–3]. Of course the Earth is an open system inextricably linked to the external world by ongoing material inputs; and as we now know, the solar system is within easy reach of billions of other habitable planetary abodes — exoplanets — in the galaxy. There is no logical requirement for life to have started on Earth.

In a public lecture by Fred Hoyle delivered in Cardiff in 1980, he expressed these views as follows:

"The very small probabilities, which one calculates for the assembly of these substances (e.g. enzymes), demonstrates as near to certainty as one would wish that life did not originate here on the Earth. Indeed, the infinitesimal probabilities demonstrate that life is even too complex for its origin to be confined within our galaxy alone. The resources of the whole universe were almost certainly needed..."

The concept of life starting *de novo* on Earth can only be defended by a *Deus ex machina* assertion thereby placing our planet in a uniquely privileged position in relation to the entire cosmos. If we adopt the premise that the requisite probability space for origination is unavailable we might be forced to adopt an anthropic argument and say: we are here on the Earth so life must have started here no matter how improbable that might be. This in essence is a religious stance and one that has become customary — indeed fashionable to adopt.

Since the discovery of DNA by Francis Crick in the 1950s combined with the discovery and sequencing of enzymes, the informational hurdle to produce life from non-life (encapsulated in Fred Hoyle's 1980 quotation) came into sharp focus. The precise ordering of nucleotides in DNA, or correspondingly of amino acids in enzymes, poses a difficulty that can only be resolved if we are permitted to extend the domain (or domains) for life's origin to encompass cosmic or even cosmological dimensions. Within such a domain of cosmic proportions the informational hurdle for starting life could be somehow overcome. Thus removing the Earth from the centre of a universal biology would constitute the ultimate Copernican revolution — the completion of a process that started over half a millennium ago.

When organic molecules were first discovered in interstellar clouds in the 1960s, it might be said that the die was already cast against the prevailing Earth-centred view of life. Contem-

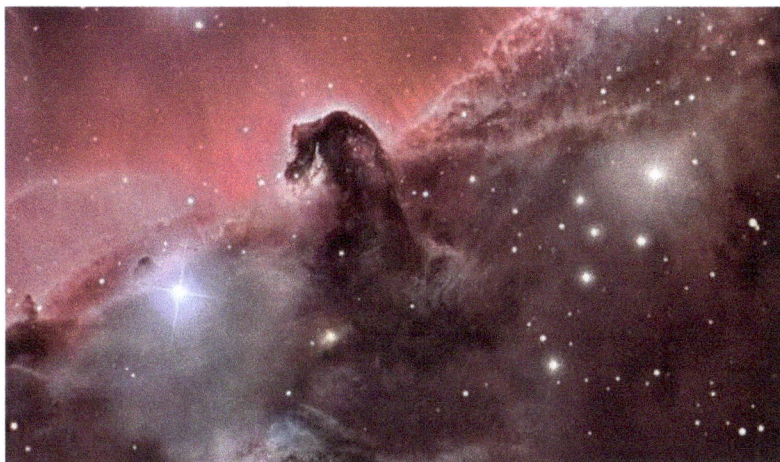

Interstellar dust cloud — the Horsehead nebula.

poraneously with the discovery of interstellar organics of ever-increasing complexity, a major paradigm shift in astronomy was being spearheaded by the authors of this book [4, 5].

At this time the strongly held astronomical opinion was that interstellar dust was comprised of ice grains that condensed in interstellar clouds. A combination of mathematical modeling and astronomical observations led to the abandonment of an ice particle model of dust giving way to a model involving mixtures of carbonaceous and siliceous dust grains. From 1974 onwards the interstellar dust was found to include a large component in the form of organic polymers — e.g. polyoxymethylene, polysaccharides, etc. [5].

In the late 1970s, when the first edition of this book was written, the time seemed right to confront the long-held view that life originated on Earth by expanding the canvas for life's origin to span the biggest available cosmological distance scales, and thereby to follow its logical consequences — one of which was diseases from space.

Laboratory evidence demonstrating the incredible space-survival attributes of bacteria and viruses were already beginning to accumulate in support of our model. We argued that once life originated in a cosmic (*not* terrestrial) setting its spread and perpetuation was inevitable. These ideas were tantamount to a revival and radical re-casting of the ancient idea of panspermia with comets playing a role in both the amplification and dispersal of life on a galactic scale [6]. If habitable planets were commonplace (which we did not know at the time, but know now) the entire galaxy will become a single connected biosphere on a relatively short time scale. The time scale could be as short as 240 Myr, the period of rotation of the solar system around the centre of the galaxy, during which a mixing of biological material between planetary systems would inevitably occur. The adoption of such a point of view regarding the astronomical origins of life would surely open up new vistas of research in astronomy as well as biology.

Supportive scientific evidence has trickled piecemeal over the past four decades from widely disparate areas of science — astronomy, biology, geology. However, each individual piece of evidence that supports the cosmic origin of life can be interpreted in a conservative manner, if one so desired, that might be seen to preserve the *status quo*. As in all past confrontations with orthodoxy the correct heterodox position must win in the long term.

The first such confrontation involved the interpretation of the interstellar extinction curve. One of us (NCW) had been working on the problem of interstellar dust for over a decade but was becoming increasingly uncomfortable with the theoretically modeling of the data with inorganic dust models [4, 5]. The fits to astronomical data were always less than perfect, and the assumptions required to obtain even imperfect fits were often arbitrary and *ad hoc*. In the late 1970s emphasis shifted to the possibility that a significant fraction of interstellar dust had a biological connotation, and with such models (after decades of failure) impressively close fits to astronomical data were possible.

One prediction of the biological model of interstellar dust was that the mid-infrared spectrum of any infrared source seen through a few kiloparsecs of dust obscuration should reveal a predicted

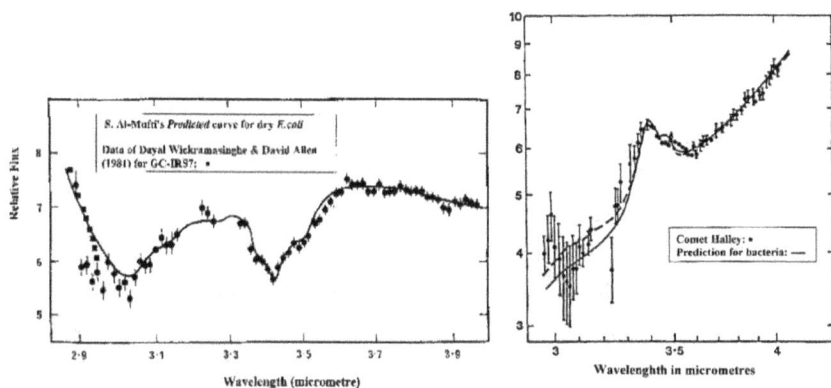

Fig. A1.1. Left panel: Comparision of the normalised flux from GC-IRS7 [6] with the laboratory spectrum of *E. coli*. Right panel: Emission by dust coma of Comet Halley observed by D. T. Wickramasinghe and D. A. Allen [7] on March 31, 1986 (points) compared with normalized fluxes for desiccated *E. coli* at an emission temperature of 320 K. The solid curve is for unirradiated bacteria; the dashed curve is for X-ray irradiated bacteria.

absorption spectrum of bacterial material. In 1982 this prediction was dramatically verified by D. A. Allen and Dayal Wickramasinghe [6]. This crucial fit that is still relevant after nearly four decades is shown in the left-hand panel of Figure A1.1.

Needless to say, this discovery and the verification of the prediction of a biological model of interstellar dust did not receive many plaudits at the time. Any dataset of this type is admittedly capable of a conservative explanation, but tediously so. A non-biological explanation of the data points in Figure A1.1 would involve *inorganically* formed organic molecules possessing functional groups that fortuitously happened to mimic biology.

A similar astronomical observation was made by the same authors (DTW and DA) for a comet, essentially yielding the same result [7]. The first infrared spectrum of a comet Comet P/Halley also showed consistency with bacterial dust emanating from an eruption of the comet in March 1986. This correspondence is shown in the right-hand panel of Figure A1.1.

More recent studies of other comets have yielded generally similar results [8]. Most recently the European Space Agency's Rosetta Mission to comet 67P/C-G has provided the most detailed observations that satisfy all the consistency checks for biology and our theory of cometary panspermia. Figure A1.2 shows the close consistency between the surface properties of the comet and the spectrum of a desiccated bacterial sample.

For many years, studies of carbonaceous meteorites have yielded evidence suggesting the presence of fossilised microbial structures [9–11]. In the early 1980s Hans D. Pflug (9) obtained what appeared to be compelling evidence of fossilised bacteria and even viruses within thin sections of the Murchison meteorite. All this data appear to have been generally ignored and never entered the mainstream of scientific discussion. Nor did later meteorite studies

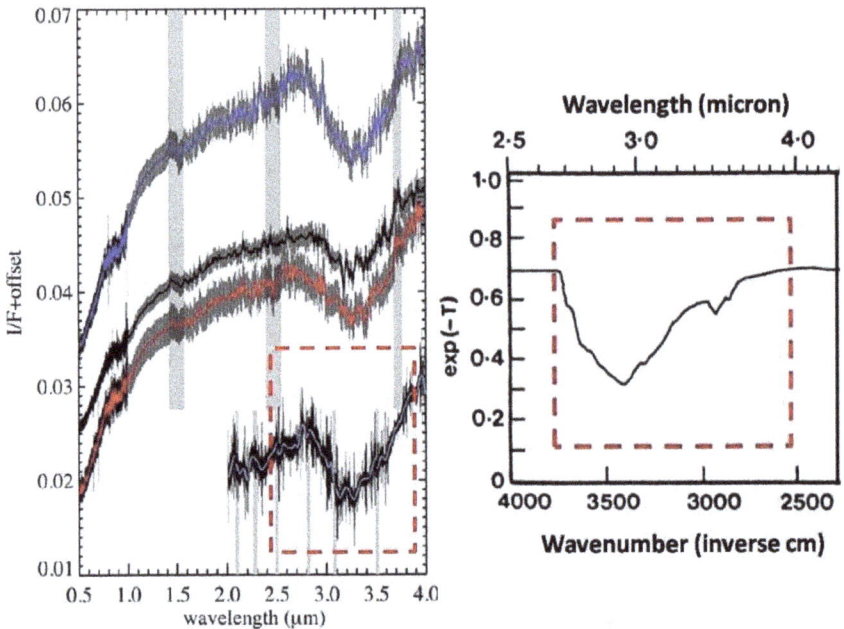

Fig. A1.2. The surface reflectivity spectra of comet 67P/C-G (left panel) compared with the transmittance curve measured for *E. coli* (right panel) (Capaccione *et al.*, 2015 (Ref. 8)).

by Richard Hoover and his colleagues working at the NASA Marshall Space Flight Centre [10]. Any meteorite "microfossil" structure is generally dismissed either as a crystallographic artifact, or contaminant. Similar refutations continued when a witnessed and recorded Sri Lankan meteorite fall in 2012 yielded even more compelling evidence of deeply embedded biological structures shown in Figure A1.3 [11]. The conservative refutation is that the stones cannot be meteorites because the signs of life within them are unequivocal. This of course would be flagrant contradiction of the reigning scientific paradigm.

Another strand in the argument is that if life came from comets in the first instance, we would expect an ongoing biological input to the Earth continuing to the present day. Is such an input

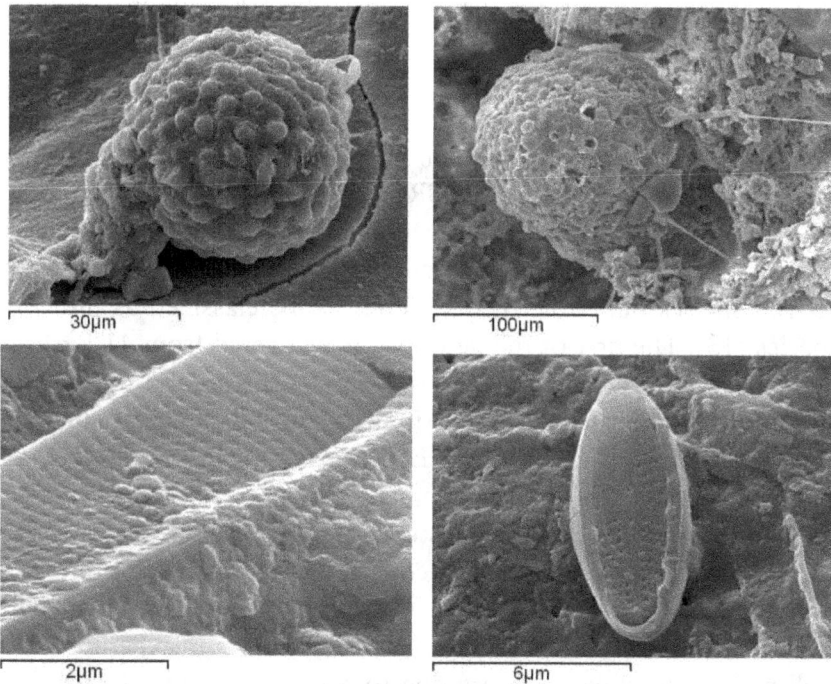

Figure A1.3.   Microfossils in the Polonnaruwa meteortite (2013). Upper frames are fossilised acritarcs extinct on Earth for billions of years; lower frames diatom frustules.

testable? From 2001 onward several balloon flights to 41 km in the stratosphere have been conducted to this end and the results have all been consistently positive [12, 13]. The implication from the stratospheric sampling of 2001 (in collaboration with the Indian Space Research Organisation) is that 0.3–3 tonnes of bacterial material (from comets) enter the Earth every day! This converts to some 20–200 million bacteria per square metre arriving from space every single day. Even this truly vast number unfortunately pales into insignificance when comparing bacteria and viruses originating from the Earth's surface some of which *could* be lofted to heights of about 3 km in upward air currents and brought down in mist and rain. The total flux of bacteria and viruses reaching heights of 3 km at the peaks of the Sierra Nevada mountains in Spain was recently measured by Reche *et al.* [14] in 2018. The average flux of mainly recycled viruses was found to be 800 million per sq m per day.

If both the space incident microorganisms and terrestrial microbes originate from disconnected pieces of a single cosmic biosphere their genetic difference may well turn out to be subtle and even difficult to detect. Indeed, an ISRO sponsored balloon flight into the stratosphere in 2006 recovered three new bacterial species that are genetically similar (80 per cent homologous) to known terrestrial species but sufficiently different to be classified as different species [13]. The first of the new species recovered from 41 km was named *Janibacter hoylei,* after Fred Hoyle, the second as *Bacillus isronensis* recognising the contribution of ISRO in the balloon experiments and the third as *Bacillus aryabhata* in honour of India's celebrated ancient astronomer.

More expensive and sophisticated investigations need to be carried out even on the samples collected so far, if we are to prove beyond doubt that these microbes are unequivocally alien. The sad truth is that funding for such vitally important experiments is well-nigh impossible to secure due to a deeply ingrained prejudice in favour of an Earth-centred theory of biology.

The Rosetta Mission to comet 67P/C-G has also revealed the comet to have a frozen surface with strong indications of subsurface liquid domains wherein microbes might be rampant [15,16]. Jets of methane and other hydrocarbons, water and molecular oxygen emerging from many locations on 67P/C-G are all consistent with biology [16]. Moreover, the material escaping from this comet examined by instruments on the ROSETTA orbiter has recently confirmed the presence of a biological amino acid glycine and high levels of H_2S and P, again pointing to biology [17].

Next we should mention that the most recent geological data places the oldest evidence of microbial life on Earth at 4.1 Byr ago, at the very beginning of the Hadean geological epoch when much of the Earth's surface was like a larva field due to the occurrence of frequent asteroid and comet impacts [18]. From what we have discussed earlier, the inference is that the impacting comets must have brought fully-fledged life.

In accordance with the scientific methodology pioneered by philosophers in the 17th century we can use the feedback loop of Figure A1.4 to generate cycles of prediction — verification — re-affirmation to put any theory or hypothesis such as ours to ever more stringent test. Needless to say, this process has led to a veritable list of successes and confirmations over the past three decades implying consistency if not absolute proof of the hypothesis of cometary panspermia.

The loop of Figure A1.4 reaffirming the panspermia hypothesis has been enormously strengthened over the past few decades. The spectroscopic identification of interstellar dust and molecules in space started in the 1970s is coming into ever sharper focus and their biochemical relevance, once vehemently contested, is now widely conceded. The trend remains, however, to assert without proof that we are witnessing the operation of prebiotic chemical evolution on a cosmic scale. If biological evolution and replication are regarded as the only reliable facts — life always generates new life — this must be so even on a cosmic scale.

One of the major criticisms that was levelled against the idea of viruses from space causing disease is implicit in the question that was often posed: "How can a virus of extraterrestrial origin know in advance of its arrival here the range of plants and animals

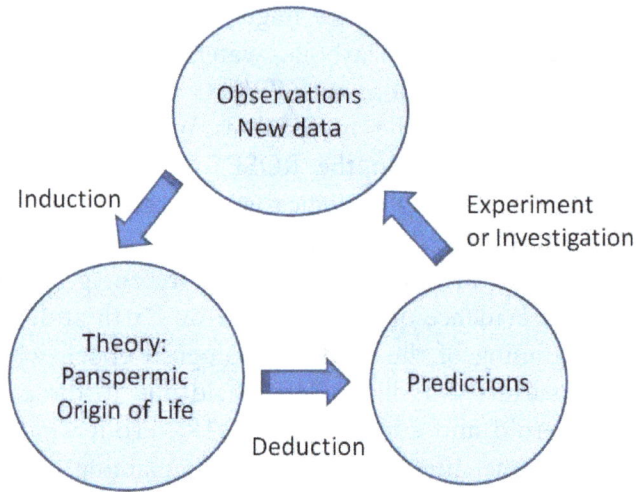

Fig. A1.4.   Inductive/deductive method of science.

with which it can interact?" In other words, viruses and their hosts would need to have an intimate connection (biologically as well as informationally) which, the argument went, would not be possible if they had originated and evolved in vastly separated cosmic venues — Earth and Space. On the face of it, it looked like a one-line disproof; but it did not take into account the history of life on the Earth and the Universe, which in our view are intimately interlinked. The footprints of viruses in the genomes of all terrestrial life forms began to be unraveled only at the turn of the millennium when whole genomes, including the human genome, came to be sequenced for the first time in 2001. One of the many surprises that followed was the discovery that what was once considered "junk DNA" actually had a viral origin. Perhaps as much as ten per cent of our DNA consists of retroviral sequences (endogenous retroviruses, ERVs) — RNA viruses that have reverse transcribed their RNA into DNA. These are the footprints of ancient viruses of cosmic origin that actually contributed to our evolution over hundreds of millions of years — and they clearly disprove the criticism that cosmic viruses cannot be the cause of pandemic disease.

On Earth a continued arrival of new bacteria and viruses must have taken place from the time when microbial life was first introduced by comet impacts. New viruses eventually succeed in becoming incorporated into the genomes of evolving lifeforms, this process continuing over billions of years of geological history. Such interaction of new viruses with evolved host species is not always harmonious, however. Throughout recorded history, we have clear evidence of a succession of pandemics of disease that have swept over the planet from time to time.

Several viral pandemics over the past two decades that have affected humans bear more than a hint of a space origin as are listed below:

Table A1.1.   Major epidemics/pandemics in the past two decades.

2019–2020	SARS-CoV2
2010–2016	Scarlet fever (Steptocossus pyogenes)
2015	Zika
2014	Ebola
2013	Influenza A/H7N9
2012	MERS
2009	Influenza A/H1N1
2002	SARS-CoV1

Of particular relevance to the world today is the COVID-19 pandemic caused by a SARS type virus (SARS-CoV1). Evidence relating to the space origin of this virus will be discussed in Appendix 3.

In the year 2020, nearly two decades after the passing away of Fred Hoye a formidable body of evidence has accumulated all pointing to life being a truly cosmic phenomenon, thus making the reigning Aristotelean concept of an Earth-centred origin of life, and indeed of diseases, look ever more flimsy. The ultimate Copernican revolution may well be just round the corner.

References

[1] Hoyle, F. and Wickramasinghe, N.C. (1980). *Evolution from Space* (J.M. Dent and Sons, London).

[2] Bieler, K., Altwegg, H., Balsiger, A. *et al.* (2015). Abundant molecular oxygen in the coma of comet 67P/Churyumov–Gerasimenko, *Nature* **526**, 678–681. doi:10.1038/nature15707.

[3] Boehnke, P., Harrison, T. *et al.* (2015). Potentially biogenic carbon preserved in a 4.1 billion-year-old zircon, *PNAS*. www.pnas.org/cgi/doi/10.1073/pnas.1517557112.

[4] Wallis, M.K. and Wickramasinghe, N.C. (2015). Rosetta images of comet 67P/Churyumov–Gerasimenko: Inferences from its terrain and structure. *Astrobiol Outreach* **3**, 12.

[5] Hoyle, F. and Wickramasinghe, N.C. (1962). On graphite particles as interstellar grains, *Mon. Not. Roy. Astr. Soc.* **124**, 417.

[6] Pflug, H.D. (1984). *Fundamental Studies and the Future of Science,* Wickramasinghe, N.C. ed. (Univ. Coll. Cardiff Press).

[7] Wickramasinghe, D.T. and Allen, D.A. (1986). Discovery of organic grains in Comet Halley, *Nature* **323**, 44–46.

[8] Hoyle, F. and Wickramasinghe, N.C. (1991). *The Theory of Cosmic Grains* (Kluwer, Dordrecht).

[9] Hoyle, F. and Wickramasinghe, N.C. (2000). *Astronomical Origins of Life: Steps towards Panspermia* (Kluwer, Dordrecht).

[10] A'Hearn, M.F. *et al.* (2005). Deep impact: Excavating comet tempel 1, *Science* **310**, 258–264.

[11] Shivaji, S. *et al.* (2009). *Int. J. Syst. Evolution. Biol.* **59**(12), 2977–2986.

[12] Hoover, R.B. (2011). Fossils of cyanobacteria in CII carbonaceous meteorites, *J. Cosmol.* **13**, 3811–3848.

[13] Wallis, J. *et al.* (2013). The Polonnaruwa meteorite: oxygen isotope, crystalline and biological composition, *J. Cosmol.* **21**, 10004–10011.

[14] Altwegg, K., Balsiger, H., Bar-Nun, A. *et al.* (2016). Prebiotic chemical — amino acid and phosphorus in the coma of comet 67P/Churyumov–Gerasimenko, *Sci. Adv.* **2016**(2), e1600285.

[15] Reche, I., D'Orta, G., Mladenov, N. *et al.* (2018). Deposition rates of viruses and bacteria above the atmospheric boundary layer, *The ISME J.* https://doi.org/10.1038/s41396-017-0042-4.

[16] Wickramasinghe, N.C., Steele, E.J., Gorczynski, R.M. *et al.* (2020). *Virol. Curr. Res.*, **4**(1). doi:10.37421/Virol Curr Res.2020.4.112.

[17] Capaccione, F. *et al.* (2015). The organic-rich surface of comet 67P/Churyumov–Gerasimenko as seen by VIRTIS/Rosetta, *Science* **347**(6220).

[18] Allen, D.A. and Wickramasinghe, D.T. (1981). *Nature* **294**, 239–260.

[19] Harris, M.J. *et al.* (2002). *Proc. SPIE* **4495**, 192

Appendix 2
The Survival of Cometary Cells and Viruses in Passing to the Earth

Comets follow highly eccentric orbits when they first approach the Sun, and small particles evaporated from their surfaces move to begin with in similar orbits. Such particles are then subject to forces that in the long term round out their orbits, ultimately converting them into nearly circular forms, like those of the planets. As well as the gravitational influences of the planets, scattering of sunlight — the Poynting–Robertson effect — is important in producing this rounding-out of the orbits. The Poynting–Robertson effect also causes a slow decrease in the average distance of a small particle from the Sun. In the long term, the particle spirals into the Sun.

For our purpose here, the micrometeorites entering the Earth's atmosphere can be thought of as being of two kinds:

(1) Those that quit their parent comets long ago, and which are now moving in nearly circular orbits close to the orbit of the Earth. (2) Those that quit their parent comets only recently, and which are still moving in highly eccentric orbits, like the orbit of Halley's comet shown in Figure A2.1.

Small particles after leaving a comet become exposed to sunlight. X-rays, ultraviolet light, and sometimes even visible light, are lethal to bacteria and viruses. Shielding against ultraviolet and visible light could easily be achieved by cometary debris, but shielding against the harder X-rays would not be possible for small particles. So unless cometary viruses and bacteria travelled in quite large clumps (as may possibly happen in some cases), they would

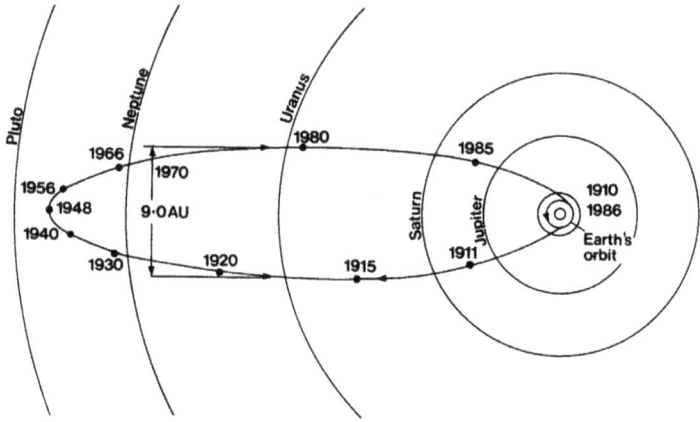

Fig. A2.1. Orbit of Halley's comet in relation to planetary orbits.

be exposed to destruction from the moment they were evaporated from the parent bodies.

The X-ray emission from the Sun is enormously variable. The X-ray flux near the Earth at the time of the large flares which occur near sunspot maximum would expose a cell, or a virus contained within a cell, to a radiation rate of about 1 Röntgen per second. At sunspot minimum, on the other hand, the radiation rate would usually be at least a million times smaller than this — i.e. less than one-millionth of a Röntgen per second. Bacteria, especially if frozen, can withstand total radiation doses in the range 10,000 to 100,000 Röntgens, whereas viruses can withstand doses upwards of 1 million Röntgens. Since the large solar flares last only for about an hour, a single big flare would not be of drastic consequence, but very many such flares would indeed be lethal to both bacteria and viruses.

Returning to the above two categories of micrometeorite, those of type (1), which have been exposed for very many years, must have become sterilised by solar X-rays. Those of type (2), however, may have spent only a few weeks or months in the inner regions of the solar system. Survival for a fraction of such particles is therefore likely, except perhaps at times around sunspot maximum.

It follows from these considerations that for maximum viability we must confine attention to bacteria and viruses that have quit their parent comets only recently, and which therefore are in highly eccentric orbits around the Sun. Exposure to solar radiation will evidently be less for newly evaporated particles on their inward journey before perihelion passage than for particles moving outwards after perihelion. The flux of such inward-moving particles is greatest in mid-winter, when the terrestrial hemisphere in which we happen to live leans away from the Sun. This orientation effect could well play a role in the seasonal incidence of diseases.

From here on we shall consider, for the reason just given, only particles moving in highly eccentric orbits around the Sun. Whereas meteoroids in the range of sizes from 0.1 to 1 cm vaporise on entering the Earth's atmosphere, giving rise to the meteors or 'shooting stars' visible to the naked eye, particles with dimensions appreciably less than 0.1 cm survive entry into the atmosphere, eventually settling to ground level.

The kinetic energy to be dissipated by a micrometeorite of mass m is $\frac{1}{2}mv^2$, where v is the speed of entry into the atmosphere. It is relevant to the time available for radiating this energy as heat whether the particle enters vertically or at a glancing angle. For vertical incidence, the time is of the order of that required to descend a scale height H, and can be taken to sufficient accuracy as $2H/v$ (i.e. descending a distance H at an average speed of $0.5v$), whereas for entry at an angle θ to the vertical the time is increased, by the factor $\sec\theta$ if the curvature of the Earth is neglected. Subject to the latter assumption, the stopping time would be $2H\sec\theta/v$, which becomes infinitely large as the angle θ tends to 90°. This infinity is not real, however. When account is taken of the curvature of the Earth, it is not hard to show that in the case of θ near 90°, the stopping time is close to $4\sqrt{RH}/v$, where R is the radius of the Earth. About 0.1 per cent of micrometeorites are involved in this extreme glancing angle situation. Although this fraction is small, it is nevertheless relevant to consider this case for obtaining the largest size that viable entering cells can have. It is also relevant that cells, once having reached the Earth, can undergo a biological multiplication in their number, so that their eventual population may have little relation to the initially incident population. Dividing $\frac{1}{2}mv^2$ by the stopping time $4\sqrt{RH}/v$ gives

$$\frac{1}{8}\frac{mv^3}{\sqrt{RH}}.$$ (A2.1)

This formula determines the rate at which energy must be dissipated from the surface of the particle.

During the moments when a particle is being violently impacted by molecules of the air, the physical properties of the surface will be much changed. There will be a large number of radiation oscillators distributed through several atomic layers, which we think should permit the surface to radiate heat at an optimum rate. Provided the particle is not too small (larger in diameter than the radiated wavelengths divided by 2π), the optimum rate is that given by the black-body formula. For a sphere of radius a this is $4\pi a^2 \sigma T^4$, where $\sigma = 5.669 \times 10^{-5}$ is the Stefan–Boltzmann constant (a is in cm, T is in degrees Kelvin, and the radiation rate in ergs per second). Equating to (A2.1), and using $m = 4\pi a^3/3$ for a particle with density close to water, leads to

$$a = 24 \cdot \frac{\sigma T^4}{v^3} \cdot \sqrt{HR}.$$ (A2.2)

We now discuss the quantities appearing on the right-hand side of (A2.2).

The constant $\sigma = 5.669 \times 10^{-5}$ is known, and so is the radius of the Earth, $R = 6.38 \times 10^8$ cm. In the glancing angle case, micro-meteorites are stopped by the atmosphere at a height of 130 to 140 km above ground level, where the scale height H is about 20 km. When v is a specified velocity, equation (A2.2) therefore relates the radius a of a spherical particle to the temperature T to which it is momentarily heated during the stopping process. The critical quantity to discuss is therefore the entry velocity v.

Micrometeorites enter the atmosphere typically at speeds of about 40 km per sec, and we shall return later to 40 km per sec as the choice for v. For the moment, however, we are concerned with the least value that can possibly be assigned to v. Subject to an upper limit for T, above which an entering cell would not survive, the least value of v determines the largest value of the radius a of a surviving cell.

Consider a micrometeorite orbit with a perihelion distance (i.e. the closest approach to the Sun) equal to the Earth's mean distance from the Sun. If the orbit is in the same plane as the Earth's orbit, and if the Earth happens to encounter the micrometeorite, the encounter speed is either about 10 km per sec or about 70 km per sec, according as to whether the micrometeorite goes around the Sun in the same sense as the Earth or in the opposite sense. The speed of 10 km per sec is the least choice for v, whereas 70 km per sec would be the largest choice for v.

A micrometeorite entering the atmosphere accelerates as it approaches due to the Earth's gravity, and it might be thought that an allowance should be made in the choice of v for this additional effect. Particles can be captured by the atmosphere, however, in more than one encounter. The first encounter must check the initial velocity of approach, leading to the particle becoming gravitationally bound to the Earth. The first encounter has the effect of making the particle a satellite of the Earth, with an orbit that is gradually degraded in further passages through the atmosphere. The choice $v = 10$ km per sec is therefore correct as a representation of the most favourable situation for a cell to enter the atmosphere without experiencing heat death. Putting $v = 10$ km per sec, $H = 20$ km, $\sigma = 5.669 \times 10^{-5}$, $R = 6378$ km in (A2.2) leads to

$$a = 4.86 \times 10^{-14} T^4 \text{ cm}, \tag{A2.3}$$

with the temperature T in degrees Kelvin.

It remains to decide on a temperature up to which living cells could survive for a time of some tens of seconds. Laboratory sterilisation procedures under dry conditions involve heating to about 425°Kelvin for an hour or more. For a sudden flash heating on a time scale about a hundred times shorter than that used in the laboratory, a survival limit of 500°Kelvin would seem reasonable.

Putting $T = 500$ K in (A2.3) gives $a = 3.04 \times 10^{-3}$ cm. Under the most favourable conditions, survival would therefore be possible for cells with radii up to about 30μ. This result is in good correspondence with the very large cells found in South Victoria Land by I. L. Uydess and W. V. Vishniac, *Extreme Environments* (ed. by M. R. Heinrich, Academic Press, NY, 1976). The cells in question were not those of individual bacteria but of colonies of bacteria living together within a common cell membrane of radius 30 to 40μ.

We turn now to the typical choice, v about 40 km per sec, representing the bulk of micrometeorites in eccentric orbits entering the Earth's atmosphere. A similar calculation to that given above leads to $a = 3.04 \times 10^{-3} \div 4^3 = 4.75 \times 10^{-5}$ cm, i.e. a radius of about 0.5μ, in good agreement with the size of micrococci.

So far we have considered only spherical particles. For a rod-shaped particle of length l and radius a we have radiation rate $2\pi a(a+l)\sigma T^4$, and a volume $\pi a^2 l$ in place of $4\pi/3\ a^3$. Neglecting a compared to l, we get

$$a = 16\frac{\sigma T^4}{v^3}\sqrt{HR}$$

instead of (A2.2). The radius of the rod is two thirds of the radius for the spherical case, i.e. $a = 0.32\mu$ for $v = 40$ km per sec, but there is no restriction on the length of the rod. This result is again in good agreement with the sizes of bacteria that were given in Table 2.1.

Consider now the effect of a single encounter of the Earth with a cloud of pathogenic micrometeorites, the encounter occurring at the typical speed of 40 km per sec. For how long will such an encounter provide an infall of the pathogen to ground level? Since the fall through the troposphere is rapid, we are evidently concerned in this question with fall to the base of the stratosphere. Violent storms can accelerate the fall locally, but it is the time of fall in still air that sets the overall duration of the attack. Figure A2.2 shows results calculated by F. Kasten (*J. Appl. Meteorology*, Vol 7, 944, 1968) for spheres of unit density falling in still air. Using a radius $r = 0.5\mu$ for micrococci, and 0.5μ also as

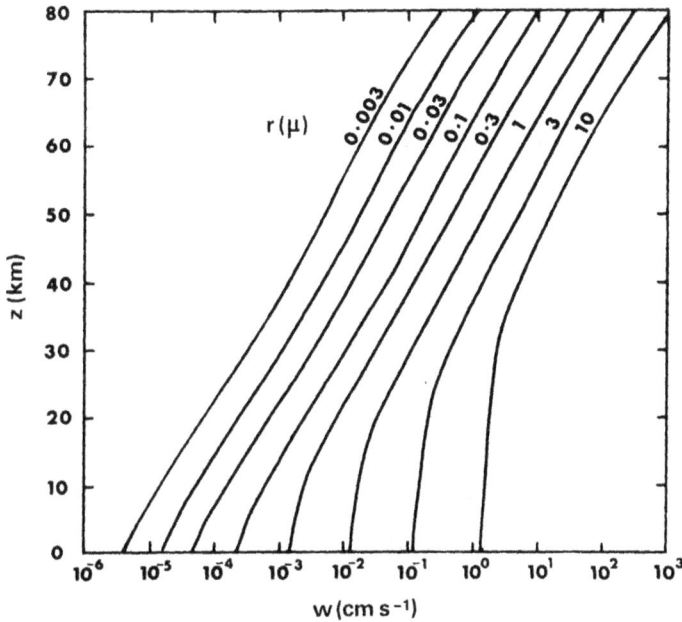

Fig. A2.2.   Falling speed of spherical particles of various radii r as a function of height z (from F. Kasten, *Journal of Applied Meteorology,* 7, 944, 1968).

a typical average dimension for rod-shaped particles, the speed of fall at a height above ground level of 15 km is seen to be about 10^{-2} cm per sec. Descent through an effective height interval of 5 to 10 km at this speed would take some two to three years. This is the general time-scale of a pathogenic attack for bacteria entering the atmosphere at about 40 km per sec, in good agreement with the time of spread of the Black Death through Europe (Figure 8.3).

The survival of a virus particle depends on its being encapsulated in some form of protective covering, and the same considerations of size and of fall time through the stratosphere apply to the virus covering as they do to bacteria.

A correlation between sunspots and influenza pandemics, shown in Figure A2.3, has recently been pointed out by Dr R. E. Hope-Simpson *(Nature,* Vol 275, 86, 1978). Solar X-ray emission

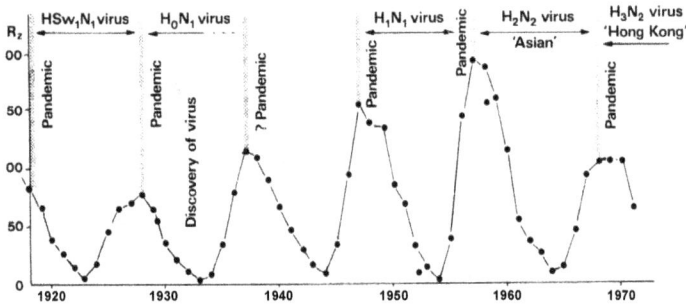

Fig. A2.3. The relation of sunspot relative numbers (Rz) to the dates of influenza pandemics (from R. E. Hope-Simpson, *Nature*, 275, 86, 1978).

depends very sensitively on the sunspot cycle and it is therefore to solar X-rays that we should perhaps turn for a connection between space-borne pathogens and the sunspot cycle. X-rays are mutagenic and might be responsible for the antigenic shifts of Figure A2.3. Displacements in timing due to the fall of virus-encapsulated particles through the stratosphere could make an actual incidence on the rising curve appear at ground level contemporaneously with the time of sunspot maximum. The coincidences of Figure A2.3 between antigenic shifts and the precise phase of sunspot maximum may therefore be somewhat fortuitous. The strongest aurorae occur at sunspot maximum. Aurorae could also be important, through electrical effects forcing the descent of small viral particles suspended in the polar regions of the stratosphere.

Over a limited number of cycles, almost any phenomenon that happens to have an approximately ten-year periodicity can be made to appear in correspondence with the sunspot curve. The symptom of false correlations is that they go out of phase as the number of cycles is increased. We ourselves had noted the apparent connection of Figure A2.3, but had become discouraged by the influenza pandemic of 1889–90, which occurred near sunspot minimum, not at sunspot maximum.

Following Dr Hope-Simpson's publication, however, we took a more detailed look at the matter, finding to our surprise that the pre-1889 situation was really quite favourable to the idea. Taking sunspot maxima from 1760 onwards, and comparing dates with those of the pandemics of Table 4.1, we have the associations of Table A2.1:

Table A2.1.

Date of Sunstlot Maximum[*]	Date of Pandemic[**]
1761	1761–62
1767	1769
1778	1781–82 (1775–76)
1787	1788–89
1804	1800–02
1830	1830–33
1837	1836–37
1848	1847–48 (1850–51)
1860	1857–58
1870	1873–75
1893	1889–90

[*]The three sunspot maxima of 1816, 1883, 1905, which do not appear in the table, were all abnormally low.
[**]Including both 'certain' and 'possible' pandemics from Table 4.1.

While the correspondences of Table A2.1 are by no means as precise as those reported by Dr Hope-Simpson, except for 1870 and 1893 the phasing is held locked to within a year or two, and this is symptomatic of a genuine connection. Furthermore, the failure at 1889–1890 is much reduced in significance, if instead of attack rates we look at the morbidity rates of Figure 4.1. These show a sudden and dramatic leap for the years 1891–1892. We believe that the 'bad' part of the influenza-sunspot association, over the years from 1870 to 1890, indicates falling off in the basic supply of the influenza virus. The situation appears to be that, if the supply of the virus is well maintained, the solar cycle modulates the severity of the disease. If on the other hand the supply dwindles to a mere trickle, then variations of the supply are more relevant than the spot cycle.

The 'English Sweats' occurred during the years from 1485 to 1552, an interval that may have some correspondence with the so-called Spörer Minimum, which lasted from about 1460 to 1550 (J. A. Eddy, *Science,* Vol 192, 1189, 1976). In the years of the Spörer Minimum there were few spots on the Sun. Possibly the causative agent of the English Sweats was very sensitive to X-rays, and so could not reach the Earth in a viable form except in a period during which there was essentially no solar activity. Possibly too the marked historical variability of diseases that we discussed in Chapter 8 may have a connection, not only with the underlying supply of pathogenic material, but also with long-term variations in the X-ray emission of the Sun.

Appendix 3
The Interpretation of Genetic Material

The double helix referred to in Chapter 10 is shown here in Figure A3.1, with its many ties of base-pairs, and is known as DNA (deoxyribose nucleic acid). The four bases are adenine (A), thymine (T), guanine (G) and cytosine (C). Each strand of the helix is an alternating chain of phosphate and deoxyribose (sugar) molecules, with a base attached to each sugar molecule, as in Figure A3.2. Thus if one considers the two phosphate molecules that are bound to a particular sugar molecule, one phosphate molecule has a CH_2 side-group attachment and the other phosphate molecule has a direct attachment to the main sugar ring, and this difference is systematically maintained along the whole chain. If we turn again to Figure A3.1 we can choose either strand and imagine going along it like a corkscrew. As each sugar molecule is encountered, will one come first to a CH_2-phosphate attachment or to a ring-to-phosphate attachment? The answer to this question depends upon which strand one chooses, because for one strand the CH_2 attachments come first at each sugar molecule, whereas for the other strand the direct ring-attachments come first. The two strands are said to have opposite polarity which are written as + and −.

Reading Figure A3.2 down the page from upper left to lower right, the bases to go with A, G, T, C cannot be arbitrarily chosen, and the following pairing rules must be obeyed. Adenine always pairs with thymine, and cytosine always pairs with guanine. These rules arise from the different sizes of the molecules and the condition that the total length of the base-pairs across the double helix must have essentially the same length, very much as the ties across a railway track must always have the same length. It is important to notice that, whereas the bases are strongly bonded to the backbone of the double helix, they are only weakly bonded to each other. This weak cross-bonding of the bases was initially of some concern to Crick and Watson when they first worked out the detailed structure of DNA, but it was then seen that the joining of the base-pairs *must* be weak. During the process whereby sex cells are produced, and also during transcription into RNA (see below), the two strands of DNA separate at the base-pairs. This separation would not be possible if the bonding between the members of each pair were strong.

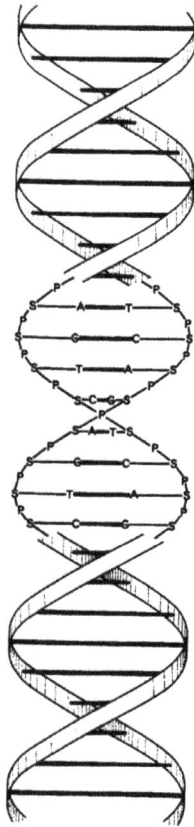

Fig. A3.1. A molecule of DNA represented as a Crick–Watson double helix.

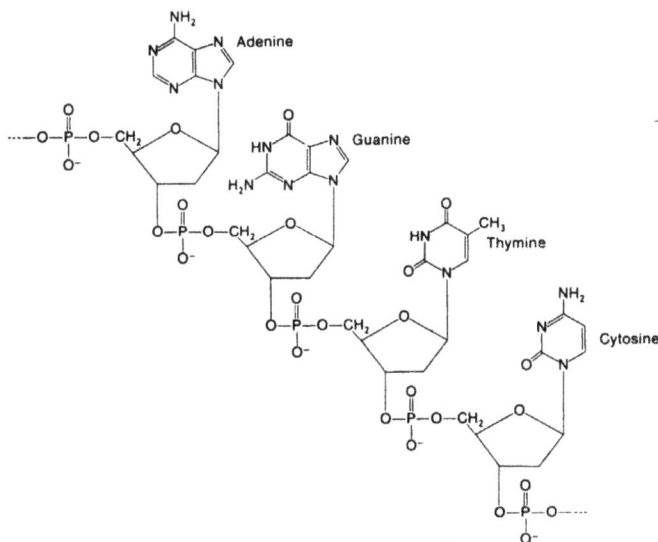

Fig. A3.2. The details of the attachments of the four bases: adenine, guanine, thymine and cytosine to the sugar-phosphate chain in DNA. A carbon atom always lies at the unmarked vertices of the ring structures. Attached to such unmarked carbon atoms there are always sufficient hydrogen atoms to make up 4 valency bonds.

DNA acts as a blueprint for the eventual production of proteins, which have the general structure shown in Figure A3.3, which R_1, R_2, ..., R_a stand for the distinctive side-chains of amino acids. Although many more than twenty amino acids can be synthesised in the laboratory, essentially only twenty amino acids appear in the proteins of life, the ones set out in Table A3.1. It is these amino acids, determining R_1, ..., R_a in the protein, that are coded for genetically by the triplets of base-pairs that we discussed in Chapter 10. Although the logic of using a base-pair triplet in DNA to determine a particular side-chain in Figure A3.3 seems simple enough, the details whereby this is actually done are highly complex. It has usually been supposed that the complex intermediate steps in DNA → Intermediate Steps → Proteins are there for the good reason that they happen to be chemically necessary to get the job

$$H_2N-\underset{\underset{H}{|}}{\overset{\overset{R_1}{|}}{C}}-\overset{\overset{O}{\|}}{C}-\underset{\underset{H}{|}}{\overset{\overset{H}{|}}{N}}-\underset{\underset{H}{|}}{\overset{\overset{R_2}{|}}{C}}-\overset{\overset{O}{\|}}{C}-\underset{\underset{H}{|}}{\overset{\overset{H}{|}}{N}}-\overset{\overset{R_3}{|}}{C}-\cdots-\overset{\overset{O}{\|}}{C}-\overset{\overset{H}{|}}{N}-\underset{\underset{H}{|}}{\overset{\overset{R_4}{|}}{C}}-COOH$$

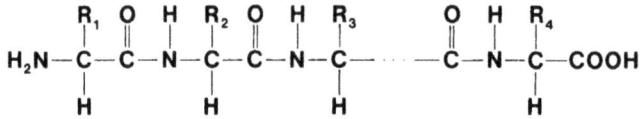

Fig. A3.3. Many linked amino acids form a protein.

Table A3.1. Amino acids.

Alanine (Ala)	Leucine (Leu)
Arginine (Arg)	Lysine (Lys)
Asparagine (Asn)	Methionine (Met)
Aspartate (Asp)	Phenylalanine (Phe)
Cysteine (Cys)	Proline (Pro)
Glutamate (Glu)	Serine (Ser)
Glutamine (Gln)	Threonine (Thr)
Glycine (Gly)	Tryptophan (Trp)
Histidine (His)	Tryosine (Tyr)
lsoleucine (Ile)	Valine (Val)

of protein production properly done. In the course of the present discussion we shall consider a very different and profound reason for the remarkable nature of the intermediate steps of protein synthesis.

A different form of genetic material is involved in the intermediate steps of protein synthesis, RNA (ribose nucleic acid). RNA is also helically twisted, but unlike DNA the RNA in terrestrial cells has only one strand — it is a single helix, with the sugar molecule ribose taking the place of deoxyribose in DNA. Bases are also attached to the ribose sugar molecules, but whereas adenine, guanine and cytosine appear as in DNA, uracil (U) replaces the thymine in DNA. The first step of protein synthesis is for an RNA transcript of the relevant gene structure on the DNA to be produced from one of the strands of the DNA. In this transcription ribose replaces deoxyribose, and uracil replaces thymine. Thus if Figure A3.2 happened to be a bit of the particular gene and of the strand under transcription, the resulting RNA would contain the corresponding bit shown in Figure A3.4. The RNA so produced then makes a journey from the nuclear region of the cell out through the cytoplasm which surrounds the chromosomes, a journey which gives the name messenger RNA (mRNA) to this first form of RNA

In the outer part of the cell there are very many nearly spherical objects with radii of about 10^{-6} cm, the ribosomes. Ribosomes contain proteins (about 40 per cent by mass), a little DNA, and a second form of RNA known as ribosomal RNA (rRNA). The mRNA travels to one of the ribosomes where a third form of RNA, transfer RNA (tRNA), is activated by the mRNA, and it is the tRNA molecules that at last do the job of putting the appropriate amino acids together into the required protein. Whereas there is an mRNA for each protein, there is a separate tRNA for each amino acid. What each individual tRNA molecule does is to associate a triplet of bases with the corresponding amino acid specified by the code of Table A3.1.

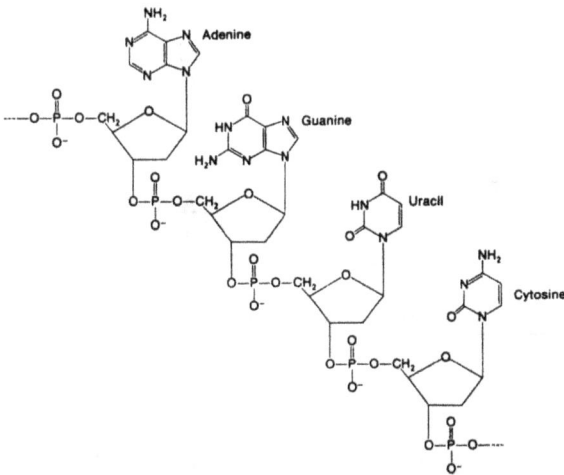

Fig. A3.4.   RNA copies one strand of DNA. This figure shows the RNA copy of Figure A3.2.

The original base-pair triplet on the DNA double helix has now coded for an amino acid through a curious sequence of steps. The triplet of base-pairs on the double helix first became a triplet of single bases, because the mRNA was transcribed from one strand only of the DNA. The triplet of single DNA bases became a triplet of mRNA bases (the same bases unless thymine was involved, in which case thymine became uracil). Next, assuming that nothing untoward occurred in the relation of mRNA to rRNA, the triplet in question gave rise to a corresponding tRNA molecule, and this tRNA molecule at last selected an amino acid according to the code of Table A3.2.

Table A3.2. The genetic code.

2nd Base / 1st Base	U	C	A	G	3rd Base
U	Phe	Ser	Tyr	Cys	U
	Phe	Ser	Tyr	Cys	C
	Leu	Ser	****	****	A
	Leu	Ser	****	Trp	G
C	Leu	Pro	His	Arg	U
	Leu	Pro	His	Arg	C
	Leu	Pro	Gln	Arg	A
	Leu	Pro	Gln	Arg	G
A	Ileu	Thr	Asn	Ser	U
	Ileu	Thr	Asn	Ser	C
	Ileu	Thr	Lys	Arg	A
	Met	Thr	Lys	Arg	G
G	Val	Ala	Asp	Gly	U
	Val	Ala	Asp	Gly	C
	Val	Ala	Glu	Gly	A
	Val	Ala	Glu	Gly	G

****Signifies chain termination.

The logic of this process goes all the way in the sense from DNA to protein, and over the past two decades this has been the habit of thinking of microbiologists. The discovery of what is known as reverse transcriptase, however, is somewhat disturbing to this way of thinking. The chemical substance which leads to DNA → mRNA is known as RNA transcriptase. Reverse transcriptase, recently found in living cells, leads to RNA → DNA. For what reason should such an inverse process exist in an entirely DNA-dominated situation?

The existence of reverse transcriptase appears to us to give support to the ideas of Chapter 10. We argued there that terrestrial plants and animals evolve by adding viruses into their genetic material. Indeed we argued that genetic material is nothing but a conglomeration of viruses and bacteria. The genetic material of viruses, however, is not always DNA. Sometimes it is RNA and sometimes DNA, sometimes double-stranded, sometimes single-stranded +, sometimes single-stranded −. To make use of all these cases, it is necessary that interconversion chemical processes should exist. Terrestrial plants and animals require reverse transcriptase in order that RNA-viruses can be added to DNA-based genetic material. Otherwise, RNA-viruses would inevitably be wasted. Evolutionary pressure towards the maximum rate of addition of new genes would therefore favour selectively the form of protein synthesis that has led to the development of reverse transcriptase.

New viral genes would probably not immediately be 'useful'. From the point of view of the host cell, they would usually code only for 'nonsense' proteins. How then could evolutionary pressures cause initially neutral genes to be changed to environmentally advantageous ones? Mistakes occur occasionally in the copying of a base pair, thereby changing the resulting protein. Such a Mendelian form of mutation of a new gene could in principle provide an answer to our question, and quite possibly the answer may be correct for the simplest life forms — bacteria and single-celled algae — for which populations and numbers of generations are both large. No such explanation can be given, however, for the emergence of the higher mammals, because for these the available time-scale is short, generations are long, and both populations and numbers of offspring per mating pair are small. The paradox of the Mendelian point of view — i.e. mutations through base-pair copying errors — is that the paleontological record shows evolution to have been dramatically rapid in precisely the case that is least favourable to such a point of view, whereas for the much more favourable case of bacteria and single-celled algae evolution was exceedingly slow.

It will be as well to illustrate these statements by numerical estimates. The chance of a detectable error occurring in the copying of a gene is usually taken to be about 10^{-6}. In a typical gene there are of the order of 10^3 base-pairs, and a copying error in many of this number would have a noticeable effect on the gene. Probably as many as 10^2 of the base-pairs would be critical in this respect. The chance of a copying error for an individual base-pair must therefore be of the order of 10^{-8}.

On the basis of these numbers, we can now enquire as to the probability of a particular triplet of base-pairs being changed through random mutations to some other specified triplet. Since the third member is often not important to the amino acid coding (see Table A3.2), it will be sufficient to consider changing only the first two members of the initial triplet, which we will suppose to be initially neutral to the survival of some animal. We shall assume the animal population to be stable, to number 10^5, and to have a generation length of 10 years.

Consider what happens to such a population in 3×10^6 years. In this span of time there are 3×10^5 generations. With 10^5 animals in each generation, it follows that 3×10^{10} animals are born in 3×10^6 years. The chance of a specified base-pair change at each birth being 10^{-8}, it is clear that after 3×10^6 years about 300 animals possess one or other of the required changes of base-pairs, which means that the chance of a particular animal possessing either change is $300 \div 10^5$. And the chance of a particular animal possessing both changes on the same chromosome is $(300 \div 10^5)^2$. Hence for a population of 10^5, the number of animals possessing both pair changes is $10^5 (300 \div 10^5)^2$, and this is close to just one animal. The time required to change only one amino acid in a specified way is therefore enormously long, and the time required to change two amino acids in specified ways would be greater than the age of the solar system. (The chance of an animal possessing one of the required base-pair changes on one chromosome and the other change on the paired chromosome is considerably larger than the number just calculated. So one might wonder if sexual cross-over could bring two such initially separated changes into the same chromosome. For animals with long chromosomes, the chance of this happening is very small indeed, however, because the cross-over would need to occur at a precisely determined place.)

We must conclude therefore that for the higher mammals random Mendelian mutations could not have shaped initially neutral genes into the many useful and dramatically effective genes that have assuredly developed among the higher mammals.

While there is general increase in the amount of DNA along the evolutionary record (typically $\simeq 10^4$ base-pairs for a virus, $\simeq 3 \times 10^5$ for a bacterium, $\simeq 3 \times 10^7$ for fungi and unicellular algae, $\simeq 10^9$ for bony fish, and $\simeq 3 \times 10^9$ for the higher mammals), the relationship between functional complexity and the amount of DNA is by no means strict. Some fish and amphibia, for example the salamander and newt, have about twenty-five times more DNA than a human (cf. J. D. Watson, *Molecular Biology of the Gene*, Chapter 17, W. A. Benjamin, 1976; S. Ohno, *Evolution by Gene Duplication*, Allen and Unwin, 1970). This great quantity is achieved, however, merely by a large-scale repetition of a comparatively small number of genes. The genes of mammals, on the other hand, usually occur only once. The mammalian DNA is used less inefficiently therefore than the DNA of amphibia.

It is an interesting speculation that this situation may be related to cometary theory, according to which comets exist in a vast halo with radius about one-tenth of a light year. Very few of the comets are in orbits that bring them to the inner regions of the solar system, and the effective lifetimes of these few are rather short. The supply of cometary viruses and bacteria would therefore disappear unless further distant comets were perturbed by passing stars into orbits that brought them to the neighbourhood of the Earth. To be effective in this respect, a passing star would need to approach to within about one-tenth of a light year of the Sun, a situation that arises about once in a hundred million years. It is likely therefore that over some geological epochs, no cometary viruses or bacteria were added at all to the Earth. In this situation, mutations would be restricted to the very slow base-pair copying errors that we considered above. Large-scale gene duplication would then be a device towards speeding the mutation rate. For N similar genes, the chance of a particular amino acid change occurring for any one of the genes would evidently be increased by N, while the number of generations required to achieve such a change would be reduced by $1/\sqrt{N}$. Even so, the evolution rate would still be very slow, which is why the salamander and newt, despite their great quantities of DNA, have never come to very much. Indeed, the amphibians are a clear demonstration of the feebleness of an evolutionary process based only on gene duplication.

How then have the new genes responsible for the evolution of the higher mammals been rendered useful? Let us return to the analogy between genes and words that we used in Chapter 10. We should think of a useless gene as a wrong word for the particular message we wish to express, not as a random jumble of letters. Thus if there are standard sequences of letters appearing in many words, like the juxtapositions 'que', 'ion', 'th', 'ing', these juxtapositions will be maintained in the initially useless gene. By the addition of more and more viruses we have at our disposal a longer and longer string of genetic letters satisfying the standard juxtapositions of genetic language. Our aim now is to produce a meaningful gene with (let us suppose) a known sequence of letters. This we do in a logically simple way. We run along the sequence of the useless genes blacking out letters until we come to the first of the required letters, and this we allow to stand. If the first required letter happened to be 'q', then 'u' will follow, as we require from standard juxtaposition, and this too we allow to stand. Sooner or later, however, we arrive at an unwanted letter, and then we continue striking out letters until once again we come to the next wanted letter. Likely enough we will come to the end of the first useless gene before we have managed to secure the full length of our wanted gene. There we shall encounter an END marker rather than a letter, but this too we shall strike out. Proceeding far enough, however, we must reach the end of our wanted gene. So by a suitable masking technique we can construct any gene we please. True the technique is likely to be wasteful of genetic material (i.e. DNA), but if we can acquire enough DNA this difficulty is overcome. From our point of view the wastefulness is advantageous, for it explains the imperative need of the higher mammals to acquire all the genetic material that has been going. Everything has been grist to the mill. At the end of Chapter 10 we mentioned the example of a type-C virus derived both from the great cats and baboons of the old world, but not from baboons of the new world. With masking techniques, similar in principle for the two species but different in detail, both great cats and baboons could evidently make appropriate use of exactly the same genetic material.

Very recently, in the last two years, it has been found that the mRNA which directs protein synthesis does indeed skip portions of the DNA strand. Figure A3.5, obtained by S. Berget, C. Moore and P. Sharp at the Massachusetts Institute of Technology, shows mRNA matched against the DNA strand from which it could in principle be represented or controlled by base-pair triplets. Yet once again the time-scales required to change an initially neutral arrangement of base-pair triplets to the required useful forms by random mutations would be prohibitively long for the higher plants and animals.

The general method described above for converting neutral genes into useful ones, fitting as it does with the evidence of Figure A3.5, and with the curious example of genetic material shared by great cats and baboons, raises a number of further questions that we shall now discuss at some length. How is the jumping on DNA achieved, and how are instructions for the jumping process passed from parents to offspring? Our answers to these questions will be based largely on general argument, although we start from an experimental situation.

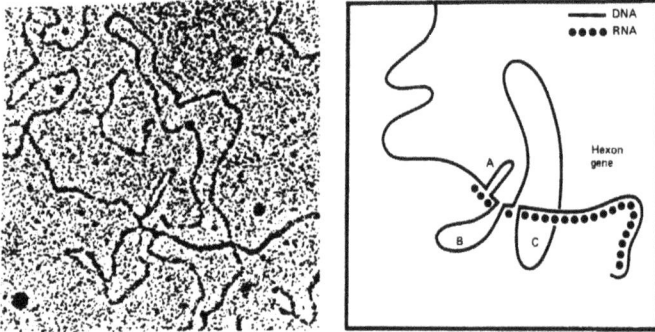

Fig. A3.5. Electron micrograph of an adenovirus mRNA molecule containing a particular gene, paired with a fragment of the viral DNA. The interpretation is that three regions of DNA (loops A, B, C) have been excluded in the RNA copy (J. Rogers, *New Scientist*, 5 January 1978, p. 18).

Transcription from DNA begins with a piece of RNA much longer than the ultimate mRNA, a piece so long that it often contains several genes (J. D. Watson, *ibid,* page 528; J. Paul in *Control Processes in Virus Multiplication,* ed. D. C. Burke and W. C. Russell, Cambridge University Press, 1978; I. M. Kerr in *Control Processes in Virus Multiplication,* ed. D. C. Burke and W. C. Russell, Cambridge University Press, 1978). It was thought formerly that this 'pre-mRNA' contained the required mRNA for each gene as a single interior segment flanked by extensive unwanted segments. It is realised now, however, that the mRNA for each gene must be constructed from several separated pieces within the pre-mRNA. The required bits of mRNA must evidently have markers of some sort to distinguish them, a marker both at the beginning and end of every wanted segment. As in editing a strip of film, we can imagine the pre-mRNA being cut at all the marker points, and the wanted segments of each gene then being spliced to give the mRNA. On further thought, however, one can see that this analogy is too facile. The human editor uses a viewing instrument to ensure that the cut pieces of film are spliced in the correct sequence. Unless we can find the equivalent in biology of a viewing instrument and of the editor's brain, the analogy fails. Otherwise cutting pre-mRNA like a film would lead to great confusion, because of ambiguity over the sequence into which the various bits should be spliced. The number of possible sequences is given by the factorial of the number of bits, which for four bits is twenty-four arrangements, of which twenty-three would be incorrect.

The film analogy is therefore quite likely to be misleading, and instead of it we can imagine a snip-and-join device going step by step along the whole of the pre-mRNA. Except over wanted segments, the device snips out units consisting of a base (A, G, U or C) together with its ribose-phosphate link on the RNA strand. Each beginning marker of a wanted segment has the property of suppressing this device, while each end marker reactivates it. Our concern here is not with the details of snipping (or of splicing) but with the nature of beginning and end markers — such markers are necessary in any system for assembling mRNA from several bits.

The markers could consist of chemical attachments to particular bases, but such attachments could move all too readily from the correct bases to other bases, giving rise to incorrect gene expression. Such a system would surely be unstable. The markers could consist of sequences of bases long enough to be sufficiently distinctive, sequence with ten to twenty bases, say. There could be one standard sequence meaning BEGIN and another meaning END. Such a system would be likely to suffer from an opposite defect, however, the defect of being much too rigidly stable. We saw above that changing only two adjacent bases was slow enough. Changing ten adjacent bases through copying errors would be impossibly rare. Such a system would be inflexible under evolutionary pressure. Indeed both these systems suffer from the further serious defect of being unspecific with respect to the particular genes under transcription. Neither could be used to control variations from one gene to another.

Another idea which has been suggested is literally to mask-out unwanted DNA segments by a surface coating of some form, or forms, of protein. While one could conceive of protein coatings being responsible for a coarse form of masking of DNA, and of being involved in the transcription of pre-mRNA, such coatings appear too imprecise to be responsible for the delicate final assembly of mRNA.

Let us return to the second of the above possibilities, of markers being represented by short sequences of bases, but not now by standard sequences. The beginning marker for a wanted segment is to be simply a few of the unwanted bases that happen to precede the segment, and likewise the end marker is to be a few of the unwanted bases that happen to follow the segment. Different segments will then in general have different markers. Along a random chain of M bases, a particular short sequence of m bases can be considered unique if $M/4^m$ is small. As an example, for $M = 10^8$ the chance of finding a particular short sequence with $m = 20$ to be also present at some other location on the chain is less than 1 in 10,000.

This shift from certain short base-sequences acting as standard markers to representing the markers by whatever base-sequences happen to be adjacent to wanted segments may seem a simple step, but it changes the most fundamental concept of microbiology, that control of a cell lies in its DNA. Control lies now in the marking base-sequences, which define the genes that the DNA is permitted to express. To use a computer analogy, the DNA is relegated to the status of backing storage, with the main programme determined by a marker code.

On this view, somewhere in the cell there must be a code catalogue that specifies the short base-sequences to be used in selecting the wanted segments of the DNA. The requirement for great precision points to chromosomal RNA as the code carrier (c.f. J. Bonner, M. E. Dahmus, D. Fambrough, R. C. Huang, K. Marushigh, and D. Y. H. Tuan, *Science*, Vol 159, 47, 1968).

Several interesting and encouraging deductions can now be made. Copying errors in such a system are of far greater consequence if they occur within the code catalogue than if they occur within a wanted segment. Such an error would have two very different effects. For the affected gene it would lead either to a wanted segment being absent from the associated mRNA, or to an unwanted segment being included in the mRNA. In either case the effect would be gross, quite unlike the minor fluctuation resulting from a copying error within a wanted segment. The second effect could be to activate some hitherto unused segment of the DNA, leading to the appearance of a quite new protein. Quite likely both the change to the old protein and the appearance of a new protein would not be helpful in an evolutionary sense, but in a small fraction of cases the resulting mutations could be a powerful stimulus to evolution.

These considerations suggest that the chance $M/4^m$ of the appearance of a new protein, following a copying error in the code catalogue, should not be too small. For $M = 10^8$ bases per chromosome, as in mammals, $M/4^m$ is of order unity for m about 13, while for $M = 10^4$, as in viruses, $M/4^m$ is of order unity for m about 7. These values of m could be optimum for evolution, being neither too small nor too large.

Assuming each gene to be in four pieces, the markers of higher plants and animals would involve about a hundred bases per gene. So the total number of bases in the whole code catalogue of some 10^5 transcribed genes would be about 10^7. With an error rate of 10^{-8} per base copy, the chance of transmitting a coding error from parent to offspring is therefore about 1 in 10. The potential evolution rate is now rapid, in our opinion sufficiently so to explain mammalian diversity, and the explosive emergence of the human species.

At a number of different places along a chromosome, DNA has identical sequences of untranscribed bases. This hitherto mysterious feature has an interesting interpretation according to the present ideas. The presence of identical markers resulting from such repeated sequences would lead to a simultaneous transcription of genes from different locations on the DNA. Particular subsets of proteins would in this way be associated together as a group, and would be capable of acting in concert with each other, a circumstance that may well explain a speculation of classical biology: that groups of genes act collectively, producing more than a simple sum of their separate effects. This case of repeated DNA sequences apart, separate genes have their own separate markers, permitting gene control to be established through a programme operating from, or through, the code catalogue.

We remarked above on the code catalogue being passed from parents to offspring. For the mammals, are there two catalogues, one from each parent? If so, what happens to the catalogues at sexual cross-over? Splitting a sensitive code would seem a tricky and dubious operation, far more so than crossing-over of the DNA alone. It seems simpler to suppose that catalogues remain intact during the production of sex cells (meiosis), and we shall conclude with this assumption, noting however that more complex situations could conceivably arise.

The system we have described, with offspring inheriting a catalogue from each parent (the female catalogue controlling the female DNA, and similarly for the male), would be subject to strong evolutionary pressure for uniformity in the marker base-sequences, but only to much weaker selection for uniformity of the sequences of bases within the genes themselves. To see how selection pressure would operate, consider the crossing of two different pure lines — a pure line being one in which the individuals are genetically uniform. Differences of marker sequences and code catalogues would not show up critically in the first generation cross, because each pure line parent would supply a code catalogue and chromosomes that were consonant with each other. The first generation cross could actually appear superior to either parental line for the reason that individuals in the first cross would have all the transcribed genes of both parents. (This behaviour might well correspond to the phenomenon of hybrid vigour.) Matings between first generation progeny would run into deleterious effects, however, because of the mismatches between code catalogues and chromosomes that would then arise in the cross-over of DNA from the two lines. For parental lines that were rather far apart, the mismatches could indeed be so severe that the second generation would not be viable at all — the first generation cross would be sterile, as in the case of the horse and donkey.

The evolutionary pressure is strongly towards species differentiation. According to our argument, the individuals which form a species have essentially the same marker sequences. Varieties of a species come from differences of the bases within the segments of DNA defined by more or less identical markers and code catalogues. We gave a computer analogy with the code catalogue representing the 'program'. Many programs can be executed on the same computer, and likewise many creatures can operate on essentially the same DNA. The dog, horse, monkey, bear and human are all tunes played on the same instrument.

Appendix 4
COVID-19 Pandemic: A Challenge For Humanity

In this book we have discussed pandemics past and present that are linked to novel biological entities — viruses or bacteria — that originated outside our planet. An idea that was once considered outrageous is beginning to seem undeniable once it is recognised that the origin and evolution of life is now to be considered unequivocally extraterrestrial rather than a purely terrestrial phenomenon. Advances in molecular biology have shown clearly that the odds against life's origin are super-astronomical, and for this reason, it is no surprise that five decades of attempts to synthesise life *de novo* in the laboratory have consistently failed [1, 2]. The alternative view is that life arose in a cosmological context and its continuation and spread is determined by processes that we can identify as "panspermia". The theory of cometary panspermia proposed by the two authors of this book implies that comets are the principal carriers, amplifiers of bacteria and viruses in the cosmos.

A cometary impact or impacts led to the commencement of life on Earth. Very recent discoveries have shown that this happened at the very first moment on Earth when life could have survived, thus leaving no time for any *in situ* life-origin event, no matter how grotesquely improbable. Detrital zircons older than 4.1–4.2 Gy, discovered in rocks belonging to a geological outcrop in the Jack Hills region of Western Australia, have been found to contain micron-sized graphite spheres with an isotopic signature of biogenic carbon [3]. The ^{12}C-enrichment found within these inclusions may thus be taken as unequivocal evidence for the existence of microbial life on Earth before 4.2 billion years ago, during the epoch of comet and asteroid impacts.

The further evolution of life on Earth — from bacteria to eukaryotes to multi-celled life, leading to plants and animals — required additional introduction of bacterial and viral genes from comets — against which Lamarckian/Darwinian selection and evolution took place over a timescale of several billion years [4, 5]. On a positive side, viruses/bacteria arriving from space promotes evolutionary progress. On the negative side they could lead to sporadic, sometimes devastating pandemics of disease and the attenuation of certain evolutionary lineages. Since the advent of modern DNA sequencing techniques which became available from 2001 we have come to realise our evolutionary history has been marked by a long series of viral pandemics that have left their mark in a large fraction of our "inert" DNA — HERV's, ERV's (retroviruses) of various kinds [6].

Samplings of the stratosphere, combined with satellite studies over the past few decades indicate that 100–300 metric tons of cosmic dust enters the atmosphere each day. We argued in Appendix 2 that although a large fraction of this influx burns up as meteors or fireballs, a significant fraction must survive, thus implying that the total amount of bacteria and viruses entering the Earth's biosphere on a daily basis would be truly enormous. Thus it would surely be foolish to maintain that we can in any way be isolated from this microbial/viral flux that must on occasion lead to epidemics and pandemics of disease.

Comets have been regarded with awe and trepidation in many ancient cultures throughout the world. Almost without exception they have been regarded as bad omens — bringers of pestilence and death. Are these beliefs to be all discarded as primitive superstitions. Perhaps not. As a life-bearing comet makes periodic orbits around the Sun, its volatile substances are progressively vaporised and dust and debris containing biological entities are released to form a cometary meteor stream with which the Earth would inevitably interact as it ploughs this debris in the course of its orbit around the Sun. This type of cometary debris contributes, in our view, to the tons of biological material that enters our planet on a daily basis.

Pandemics Past and Present

As we have already discussed in Chapters 3 and 4, reports of the sudden spread of plagues and pestilences punctuate human history over thousands of years. The various epidemics that have been recorded often bear little or no resemblance to one another. However, they share a common property of afflicting entire cities, countries or even widely separated parts of the Earth in a matter of days or weeks. The Greek Historian Thucydides describes the *Plague of Athens* of 429 BC thus:

> "It is said to have begun in that part of Ethiopia above Egypt ...
> On the city of Athens it fell suddenly, and first attacked the men in Piraeus; so that it was even reported by them that the Peloponnesians had thrown poison into the cisterns..."

Thucydides writes that many families were simultaneously struck by a disease with a combination of symptoms hitherto unknown. The idea of an enemy (the Spartans) poisoning the drinking water rings similar to what has happened in the corona virus outbreak in China where thousands of people were infected in a couple of days.

Very similar descriptions of a sudden onset and rapid global spread is relevant to almost all earlier as well as later epidemics. Extreme swiftness of transmission is hard to comprehend if, as is usually supposed, infection can pass only from person to person. Such explanations are particularly untenable for the many epidemics that occurred before the advent of air travel when movement of people across the Earth was a slow and tedious process.

One important piece of historic evidence that emerged 101 years ago relates to the great Influenza pandemic of 1918–1919 that caused some 20–30 million deaths worldwide. Reviewing all the available data Dr L. Weinstein wrote as follows:

"Although person-to-person spread occurred in local areas, the disease appeared on the same day in widely separated parts of the world on the one hand, but on the other, took days to weeks to spread relatively short distances. It was detected in Boston and Bombay on the same day, but took three weeks before it reached New York City, despite the fact that there was considerable travel between the two cities. It was present for the first time at Joliet in the State of Illinois four weeks after it was first detected in Chicago, the distance between those areas being only 38 miles..."

L. Weinstein, *New Eng. J. Med., May 1976*

The lethal second wave of the influenza pandemic of 1918 thus showing up on the same day in Boston and Bombay defies the realities of human travel at the time. Before the advent of air travel so it was impossible for people to transfer the virus from Boston to Bombay or vice versa. Over the following months the infective agent probably became dispersed through the troposphere and came down with an expected seasonal modulation across much of the world.

The general belief, that is by no means well-proven, is that major pandemics, such as influenza as well as the present Coronavirus pandemic, start by random mutation or genetic recombination of a virus or bacterium that is already on Earth, and which then spreads across a susceptible population solely by direct person-to-person contact. The facts relating to past as well as ongoing pandemics rarely accord with such a model.

Deep Minimum in the Sunspot Cycle No. 24

In two publications in 2017 and 2019, I collaborated with a team of colleagues to point out that the Sun was approaching the deepest minimum in its cycle of sunspots in late 2019 in over a hundred years (see Figure A4.1) [9, 10]. This, in turn, implies a reduction in the flow of high-speed electrons streaming out from the Sun that serves to maintain a protective sheath of magnetic field called the magnetosheath around the planet. With a weakened magnetic

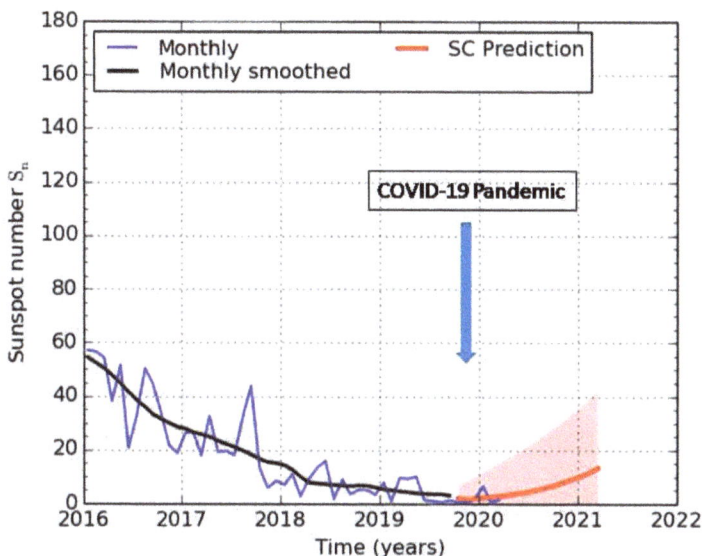

Figure A4.1.   Graph presenting the Sun approaching the deepest minimum in its cycle of sunspots in late 2019 (data from http://sidc.be/sulso-Royal Observatory Belgium).

field, our planet would consequently be more "open" to the ingress galactic cosmic rays (GCR's) as well as of charged "dust" particles from comets including bacteria and viruses from outside. On this, we warned of the risk of impending future pandemics in the foreseeable future.

An indication of such an increased ingress of virus-sized dust appears evident in the greatly enhanced frequency of noctilucent clouds that have been recorded throughout 2018 and 2019. Noctilucent clouds (NLC's) are tenuous cloud-like structures that show delicate filigree patterns visible after sunset against a not-yet-darkened evening sky. They are seen predominantly during the summer months in the latitude range 50° to 70°, both north and south of the equator, and are visible shortly after sunset during the period of astronomical twilight. In January 2020, noctilucent clouds were seen over Macquarie Island (9.8°S) and in March 2020, they were seen in the US as far south as Freedom, Oklahoma (+36°N) thus breaking all the normal rules of latitude limitation for the occurrence of noctilucent clouds https://spaceweatherarchive.com/2020/03/26/noctilucent-clouds-over-the-south-pacific/.

A dramatic picture of the distribution of NLCs on 12 June 2019 was captured by cameras onboard NASA's Aeronomy of Ice in the Mesosphere satellite (Figure A4.2). This image is a clear demonstration of the existence of a vast amount of comet/meteoroid dust of viral sizes at heights of 80 km around which ice has condensed. If this is contained in a cloud of viruses including the corona virus which found ingress into the jet stream (northern subtropical jet stream) the first cases of 2019-nCoV infection in humans reported in China during November 2019 might be explained.

It is also interesting to note that the first cases of the new Corona virus followed remarkably close on the heels of a cometary bolide that exploded on 11 October 2019 that lit up the midnight skies above north-east China in the province of Jilin.

My colleagues and I have discussed the possibility of the space origin of the Coronavirus in a series of recent papers [12–14]. My collaborator on this project, geneticist and immunologist Professor Edward Steele has analysed the gene sequences of the viruses from cases in Wuhan China and the USA and concluded that an animal transfer model is ***not viable.*** It seems to be the generally presented a *fait accompli* in the absence of any compelling evidence. So, if one is stuck with Earth-centred theories, the conclusion is that the origin of the new virus is *unknown.* However, the epidemiology of the COVID-19 pandemic that has been unravelled between November 2019 and May 2020 shows clearly all the hallmarks of a virus from a cometary source.

The data suggests that a fragile cometary bolide perhaps several metres in diameter, containing the virus, gained ingress as a dispersed particulate cloud into the northern subtropical jet stream sometime during the middle of 2019 (Figure A4.3).

The constituent particles are then quickly spread at speeds of 250 miles per hour globally throughout the jet stream. The subsequent history of the COVID-19 pandemic can be traced as

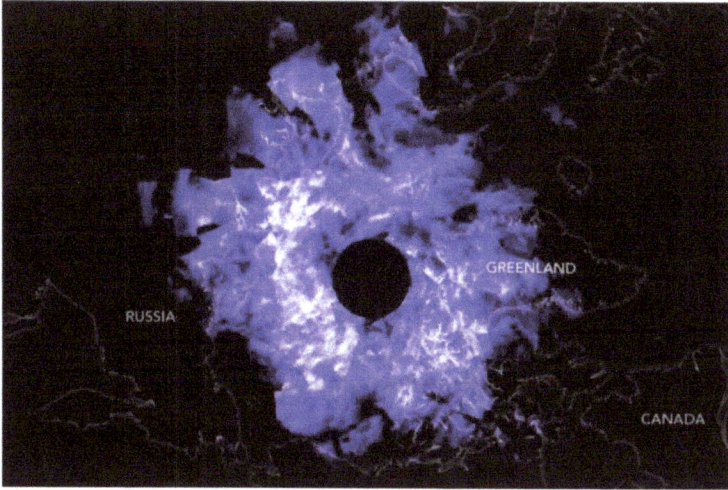

Fig. A4.2. Visible light reflected from noctilucent clouds on 12 June 2019, taken by cameras aboard NASA's AIM satellite, showing noctilucent clouds stretching far south (Courtesy NASA).

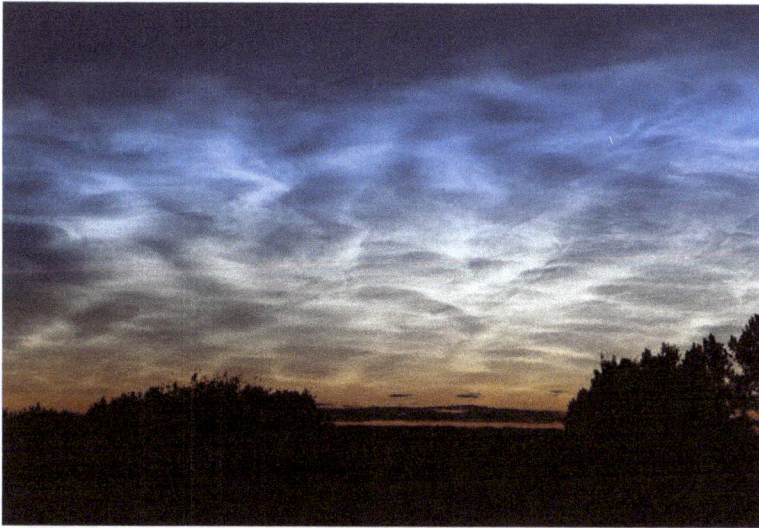

Fig. A4.3. Noctilucent clouds from the ground (Courtesy NASA).

a climatically determined breakthrough from the jet stream to ground level. As often happens (in the view expressed in this book) the mountain range of the Himalayas provides a "vulnerable" channel eastward of its high peaks for breakthrough from the troposphere. This in our view is how the first sudden and major outbreak occurred in China over a very short time. Subsequent fall-out events from the jet stream occurred over the next several months around the world. The major foci of the disease as it appeared around the globe are at locations between 30° and 50° N, all of which lie vertically below the "infected" jet stream (see Figures A4.4 and A4.5). The epidemiology of the pandemic can be explained broadly in terms of two processes: (a) primary fall-out of the infective agent leading to an exponential rise in case numbers; followed by slow person-to-person and community spread. Community spread remains an ill-defined process at the moment with many conflicting theories as to whether or not the virus can persist in viable form in dust that can circulate near ground level.

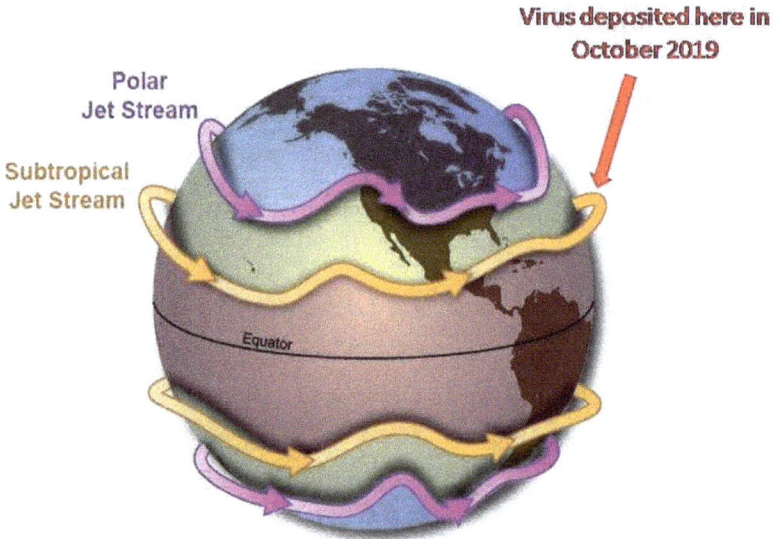

Fig. A4.4.   Jet streams straddling Earth.

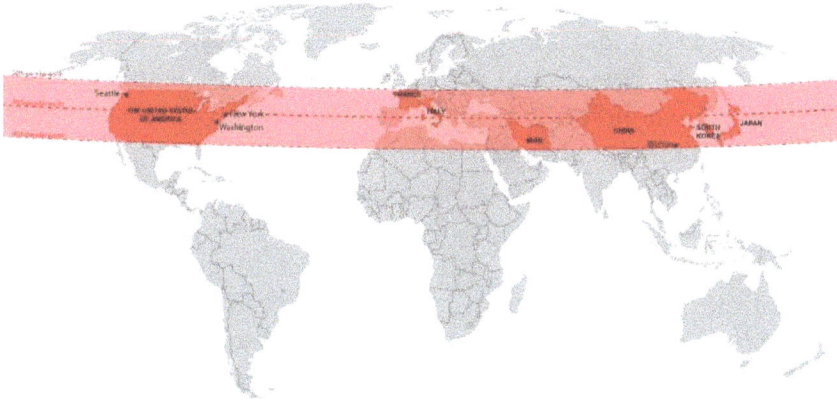

Fig. A4.5. Latitude belt of initial foci of COVID-19 virus fall-out.

Subsequent foci of COVID-19 outbreaks have developed along a narrow belt latitude 40°–60° N, with person-to-person transmission aggravating its spread within individual foci which seem to represent locations of new fall-out of the viruses.

The spread of COVID-19 in the past months is looking similar in many respects to the patterns of spread seen during the 1918–1919 influenza pandemic. Let us hope that the reservoir of the COVID-19-causing virus, if it came from the stratosphere, eventually becomes exhausted and together with the containment/social distancing measures in force, the pandemic will come to an end.

Concluding Remarks

I believe that in 2020 we have reached a crucial turning point in the history of human civilization. When it is finally accepted that life on Earth is a minuscule part of a vast cosmic biosphere, the implications for humanity will undoubtedly be profound and far-reaching. Even more important would be the recognition that alien life in the form of microbes — bacteria and viruses — exist in our midst *even now* and are continually raining down on our planet. Such microbial entities could be responsible for devastating pandemics as in the case of the COVID-19 pandemic; but more positively we should recognise that cosmic viruses and bacteria could have the potential to augment our genomes — the genomes of all terrestrial lifeforms — and over long periods unravel an ever-changing panorama of cosmic life.

The world is changing at an astonishing rate — a cliché, but true. The large subset of the changes that are distinctly for the worse are wrought by an insatiable desire to gain ever greater control of the Earth's diminishing resources, insatiable greed, and thereby to reassert our role as the supremely dominant — indeed indomitable, species on the planet. In the quest for such illusory glory we are inevitably destroying the richness and diversity of life on Earth — plants, animals, microbiota — that has been established over millions of years. Whilst advances in technology continue at an accelerating pace, humanity as a whole is becoming ever more fractured, ever more bereft of moral principles that could preserve the best in our culture. Wars and bitter sectarian conflicts and heart-rending suffering are to be seen everywhere. The "climate-change" marches and protestations of young people that are gaining momentum are perhaps emblematic of a desire to rebel against reigning paradigms that seem to be threatening our very existence.

Thomas Kuhn famously declared "...when paradigms change, the world changes with them." One could perhaps assert that a reversal of this causality is also possible — "when the world changes paradigms can be forced to change."

References

[1] Bell, E.A., Boehnke, P., Harrison, T. *et al.* (2015). Potentially biogenic carbon preserved in a 4.1 billion-year-old zircon, *PNAS*. www.pnas.org/cgi/doi/10.1073/pnas.1517557112.

[2] Deamer, D. (2012). *First Life: Discovering the Connections between Stars, Cells and How Life Began* (Univ. Calif. Press).

[3] Wickramasinghe, C. (2013). Simulation of Earth-based theory with lifeless results, *BioScience* **63**(2), 141.

[4] Steele, E.J., Al-Mufti, S., Augustyn, K.A., Chandrajith, R., Coghlan, J.P., Coulson, S.G. *et al.* (2018). Cause of Cambrian explosion — Terrestrial or cosmic? *Prog. Biophys. Mol. Biol.* **136**, 3–23. https://doi.org/10.1016/j.pbiomolbio.2018.03.004.

[5] Steele, E.J., Gorczynski, R.M., Lindley, R.A., Liu, Y., Temple, R., Tokoro, G., Wickramasinghe, D.T. and Wickramasinghe, N.C. (2019). Lamarck and panspermia — On the efficient spread of living systems throughout the cosmos. *Prog. Biophys. Mol. Biol.* **149**, 10–32. pii: S0079-6107(19)30112-9. https://doi.org/10.1016/j.pbiomolbio.2019.08.010.

[6] Wickramasinghe, N.C. (2013). DNA sequencing and predictions of the cosmic theory of life, *Astrophys. Sp. Sci.* **343**, 1–5 (arXiv:1208.5035).

[7] Pflug, H.D. (1984). *Fundamental Studies and the Future of Science*, in Wickramasinghe, N.C. ed. (Univ. Coll. Cardiff Press).

[8] Wickramasinghe, N.C., Wallis, J. and Wallis, D.H. (2013). Panspermia: Evidence from astronomy to meteorites, *Mod. Phy. Lett. A* **28**(14), 1330009.

[9] Wickramasinghe, N.C., Steele, E.J., Wainwright, M. *et al.* (2017). Sunspot cycle minima and pandemics: A case for vigilance? *J. Astrobiol. Outreach*, **5**, 2.

[10] Wickramasinghe, N.C., Wickramasinghe, D.T., Senanayake, S. *et al.* (2019). Space weather and pandemic warnings? *Current Sci.* **117**(10), 1554.

[11] Wickramasinghe, N.C., Steele, E.J., Gorczynski, R.M.. Temple, R. *et al.* (2020). Predicting the future trajectory of COVID-19, *Virol. Curr. Res.* **4**, 1.

[12] Wickramasinghe, N.C., Steele, E.J., Gorczynski, R.M., Temple R. *et al.* (2020). Comments on the origin and spread of the 2019 Coronavirus, *Virol. Curr. Res.* **4**, 2.

[13] Wickramasinghe, N.C., Steele, E.J., Gorczynski, R.M., Temple, R. *et al.* (2020). Growing evidence against global infection-driven by person-to-person transfer of COVID-19, *Virol. Curr. Res.* **4**, 3.

Index

www.ingramcontent.com/pod-product-compliance
Lightning Source LLC
Chambersburg PA
CBHW050554190326
41458CB00007B/2039